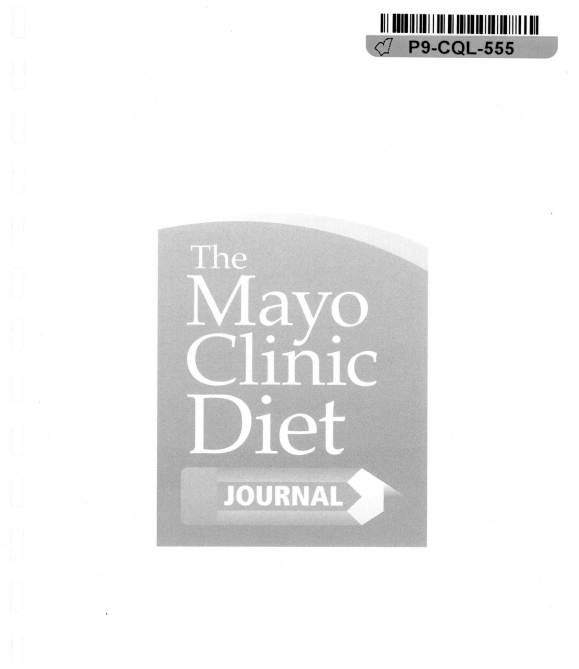

The Mayo Clinic Diet

JOURNAL

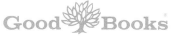

Good Books

Intercourse, PA 17534 • 800-762-7171 • www.GoodBooks.com

P9-CQL-555

# Mayo Clinic

**MEDICAL EDITOR-IN-CHIEF**
Donald Hensrud, M.D.

**ASSOCIATE MEDICAL EDITOR**
Jennifer Nelson, R.D.

**SENIOR DIRECTOR,
CONSUMER PRODUCTS & SERVICES**
Nicole Spelhaug

**EDITOR-IN-CHIEF, BOOKS AND NEWSLETTERS**
Christopher Frye

**MANAGING EDITOR**
Kevin Kaufman

**CREATIVE DIRECTOR**
Daniel Brevick

**ART DIRECTORS**
Stewart Koski, Paul Krause

**ILLUSTRATOR**
Kent McDaniel

**PROOFREADERS**
Miranda Attlesey, Donna Hanson

**ADMINISTRATIVE ASSISTANTS**
Beverly Steele,
Terri Zanto Strausbauch

Each of the habits in *Lose It!* has been the subject of scientific studies that support its role in weight management. In addition, Mayo Clinic conducted a two-week program to test the validity of this habit-based approach to quick weight loss. The 33 women who completed the program lost an average of 6.59 pounds, with individual results varying from 0.2 to 13.8 pounds lost. The 14 men who completed the program lost an average of 9.97 pounds, with individual results varying from 5.2 to 18.8 pounds lost. Individual results will vary. Consult your doctor before starting any diet program.

# Good Books

**PUBLISHER**
Merle Good

**EXECUTIVE EDITOR**
Phyllis Pellman Good

**ASSISTANT PUBLISHER**
Kate Good

Published by Good Books

All rights reserved. No part of this book may be reproduced or used in any form or by any means, electronic or mechanical, including photocopying and recording, or by any information storage and retrieval system, without permission in writing from the publisher, except by a reviewer, who may quote brief passages in review.

© 2010 Mayo Foundation for Medical Education and Research

ISBN 978-1-56148-677-9

First Edition

If you would like more copies of this book, contact Good Books, Intercourse, PA 17534. 800-762-7171. *www.GoodBooks.com.*

For bulk sales to employers, member groups and health-related companies, contact Mayo Clinic Health Solutions, 200 First St. SW, Rochester, MN 55905, or send an email to *SpecialSalesMayoBooks@mayo.edu.*

*The Mayo Clinic Diet* is intended to supplement the advice of your personal physician, whom you should consult regarding individual medical conditions. MAYO, MAYO CLINIC and the Mayo triple-shield logo are marks of Mayo Foundation for Medical Education and Research.

Photo credits: Artville, Jordan Eady and Photodisc

Cover design by Paul Krause

Printed in the USA

# Table of contents

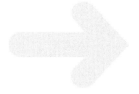

Throughout the journal you'll find this symbol, which refers you to pages
in *The Mayo Clinic Diet* book for more in-depth information.

# Welcome to *The Mayo Clinic Diet Journal* — a practical, easy-to-use resource that supports *The Mayo Clinic Diet*

You may associate a food and activity journal with lots of busywork but very little support or follow-up.

*The Mayo Clinic Diet Journal* intends to be something different. The journal guides you through the first 10 weeks of *The Mayo Clinic Diet* in clear steps. You use simple forms to compile food and exercise records each day. In addition, the journal draws on your natural abilities to:

**Learn from previous experience.** Evaluate how you did from the previous weeks in weekly reviews and reflect on what you can do to improve your program.

**Plan for the week ahead.** A series of special planning tools helps you stay on track and allows you to adjust your program — based in part on what you've learned from the reviews.

These features combine to make losing weight more personal, pleasurable and, ultimately, more successful. What you learn about yourself during 10 weeks of journal use can carry over into a lifetime of good health and healthy weight.

Here's a summary of the organization and practical tools you'll find in *The Mayo Clinic Diet Journal.*

## ❶ Get Started

Start the journal — and *The Mayo Clinic Diet* — by checking your motivations to lose weight. If you feel motivated and ready, then pick a start day and the weight goal you'd like to reach.

## ❷ Weight Record

Enter your weight from weekly weigh-ins with this tool and track how much weight you've lost from your start day. Continually update the Weight Record while using the journal.

## ❸ *Lose It!* Journal

This section organizes the initial two-week, quick-start portion of *The Mayo Clinic Diet.*

### Habit Tracker

Check boxes in the Tracker to follow your progress with the Add 5, Break 5 and Adopt 5 bonus habits of *Lose It!* Update the Tracker daily.

## Daily Record

Record everything you eat and everything you do from day 1 through day 14 of *Lose It!* Daily goal setting helps keep you motivated and engaged.

## Review

Assess your performance in *Lose It!* and prepare for the transition to the next stage of *The Mayo Clinic Diet*.

## ④ *Live It!* Journal

This section guides you through the next stage of *The Mayo Clinic Diet*. Use these tools in each weekly unit for the next eight weeks:

## Planner

At the beginning of each week, organize your schedule and plan ahead for upcoming activities.

**Week At A Glance.** Create a general overview of the coming week by scheduling meals, exercise time and other activities.

**Meal Planner.** Analyze meals to check how well they fit with your pyramid servings goals. Using this tool is optional but helpful.

**Menu & Recipe.** Refer to a sample menu each week to help guide or inspire your menu decisions.

**Shopping List.** Compile a list of food items to buy from the grocery store as you plan menus for the week ahead.

## Daily Record

Record everything you eat and everything you do — just as you did in *Lose It!* — but now include the number of pyramid servings in addition to the amounts.

## Review

At the end of each week, assess your progress and review what may have worked well and what didn't work well from the previous week. Consider how to adjust and improve your program.

# My motivation to lose weight

There may be many reasons why you want to lose weight. It's critical that you're physically and emotionally prepared for the effort. Take time to consider your motivations and the reasons why they matter. **SEE PAGE 13 OF *THE MAYO CLINIC DIET.***

**MOTIVATION:**

Why it matters:

**MOTIVATION:**

Why it matters:

**MOTIVATION:**

Why it matters:

**MOTIVATION:**

Why it matters:

# My starting point

What's going on in your life right now? Are you motivated? Are your weight goals realistic? Will family and friends support you? Now may be a good time to start *The Mayo Clinic Diet.* 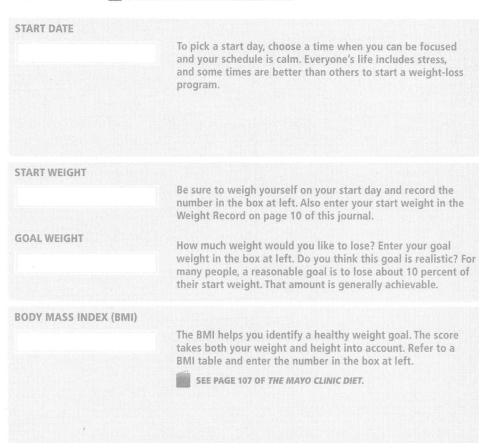 SEE PAGE 15 OF *THE MAYO CLINIC DIET.*

**START DATE**

To pick a start day, choose a time when you can be focused and your schedule is calm. Everyone's life includes stress, and some times are better than others to start a weight-loss program.

**START WEIGHT**

Be sure to weigh yourself on your start day and record the number in the box at left. Also enter your start weight in the Weight Record on page 10 of this journal.

**GOAL WEIGHT**

How much weight would you like to lose? Enter your goal weight in the box at left. Do you think this goal is realistic? For many people, a reasonable goal is to lose about 10 percent of their start weight. That amount is generally achievable.

**BODY MASS INDEX (BMI)**

The BMI helps you identify a healthy weight goal. The score takes both your weight and height into account. Refer to a BMI table and enter the number in the box at left.

SEE PAGE 107 OF *THE MAYO CLINIC DIET.*

**WAISTLINE MEASUREMENT**

To determine whether you're carrying too much weight around your middle, use a flexible tape and measure around your body just above the highest points on your hipbones. Record your results in the box at left.

SEE PAGE 108 OF *THE MAYO CLINIC DIET.*

## The Mayo Clinic Diet

Have questions about some of the basics of your weight-loss program? You may find answers in *The Mayo Clinic Diet* book.

Common questions that you may have about eating healthy, being active and losing weight are organized in the list at right. The page numbers accompanying each question cross-reference material in *The Mayo Clinic Diet* book that may provide you with answers.

## Basics

| | |
|---|---|
| What is the Mayo Clinic Healthy Weight Pyramid? | 18, 122-131 |
| What is my healthy weight? | 104-111 |
| What is my daily calorie goal? | 69 |
| What are my daily serving recommendations? | 71 |
| How much is in a serving? | 71-73, 80-89 |

## Healthy eating

| | |
|---|---|
| How do I create a weekly menu? | 76-79 |
| What are healthy shopping strategies? | 158-159 |
| What are the serving sizes of different foods? | 208-235 |
| How do I overcome barriers to healthy eating? | 181-189 |

## Activity and exercise

| | |
|---|---|
| How do I start exercising? | 30-31, 50-51 |
| How many calories do I burn when I'm active? | 179 |
| How do I increase the amount of activity I do? | 50-51, 96, 175 |
| How do I set up a good exercise program? | 94-95, 173,174 |

## Behaviors

| | |
|---|---|
| How do I set goals? | 54-55, 66-68 |
| How do I change a behavior? | 132-141 |
| How can I stay motivated? | 13-14, 16-17, 149 |
| What can I do when I slip up? | 142-155 |

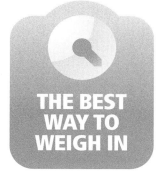

## THE BEST WAY TO WEIGH IN

With *The Mayo Clinic Diet*, you'll weigh yourself at least once a week. Record the results in your Weight Record.

→

How regularly should you weigh yourself? That depends. Checking the scale too often can cause you to obsess over minor daily weight changes. Not checking enough may indicate that you're not focused and involved with your weight program.

A good rule of thumb is to weigh yourself about once a week. If you feel a need to do so more often — several times a week or even daily — that's OK. Just remember that the long-term weight trends occurring over weeks or months are generally more important to know than are day-to-day changes.

Be consistent with your weigh-ins from week to week. Schedule them on a regular day and at a regular time and try to stick with that routine. Along with providing more uniform results in your Weight Record, consistency also helps to keep you engaged in your weight-loss program.

You'll need to weigh yourself on your start day of *The Mayo Clinic Diet*. It's important that you enter your start weight at two places in the journal:

✔ Weight Record (page 10)

✔ Day 1 of the Daily Record (page 18)

Later, you'll be reminded on the seventh day of each week to weigh yourself and record the weight in your Daily Record. You'll also continue to update and chart your progress in the Weight Record.

Use weigh-ins to review your progress. Be sure to reward yourself when you meet your weight goals. If you don't meet your goals, don't be too hard on yourself. Identify factors that may have worked against you and consider how to avoid them.

# Weight Record

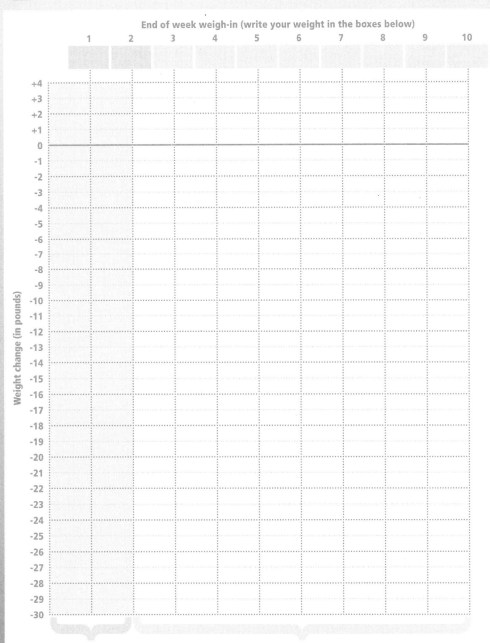

End of week weigh-in (write your weight in the boxes below)

| | 1 | 2 | 3 | 4 | 5 | 6 | 7 | 8 | 9 | 10 |
|---|---|---|---|---|---|---|---|---|---|---|

Weight change (in pounds)

+4
+3
+2
+1
0
-1
-2
-3
-4
-5
-6
-7
-8
-9
-10
-11
-12
-13
-14
-15
-16
-17
-18
-19
-20
-21
-22
-23
-24
-25
-26
-27
-28
-29
-30

Lose It!          Live It!

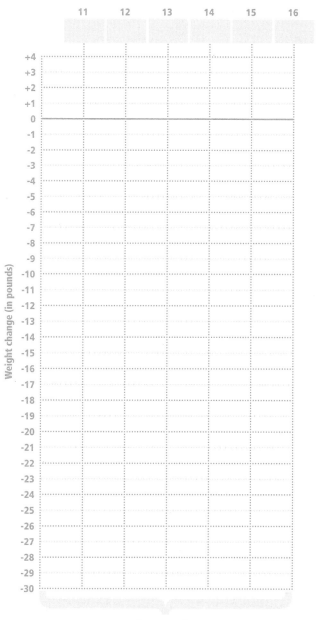

**DIRECTIONS:**

1. Write your start weight in the box at the top of the page.

2. After each weekly weigh-in, write your current weight in the box under the appropriate week.

3. Subtract your current weight from your start weight to calculate your weight change.

4. Mark your weight change for each week on the table.

5. Connect the marks to form a line graph of your progress.

# Lose It!

This section of *The Mayo Clinic Diet Journal* is designed to help you safely lose 6 to 10 pounds in two weeks and jump-start your weight loss. It's easy to get started.

# How to record *Lose It!*

**1** Start each day by setting a realistic, achievable goal in the Daily Record.

**2** Record the amount of time you spend doing exercise and being active. Activity should be moderately intense and sustained for five minutes or more.

**3** Record everything you eat during the day, including amounts (in most cases, your best estimate will do).

**4** At the end of each day, mark the Habit Tracker to indicate which of the Add 5, Break 5 and Bonus 5 habits you successfully achieved.

**5** Following day 7 and day 14, total the rows and columns of the Habit Tracker. This may help you identify problems and improve your program.

**6** Following day 14, use the Review to assess your progress in *Lose It!* and prepare for your switch to *Live It!*

---

## Lose It!

**DAILY RECORD • DAY 5**

**DAY 5**

**1** TODAY'S GOAL:
add 10 extra minutes of exercise to my walking routine!

**2** TODAY'S ACTIVITIES:

| | Time |
|---|---|
| early morning walk | 10 minutes |
| walk during lunch break | 10 minutes |
| water aerobics class | 30 minutes |
| yardwork | 15 minutes |
| **Total time (in minutes)** | 65 minutes |

**MOTIVATION TIP:**
Learning to say no to things that aren't essential gives you time for things you really want to do.

**3** WHAT I ATE TODAY:

| Time | Food item | Amount |
|---|---|---|
| 7:00 | cereal | 1 cup |
| | grapefruit | half |
| | milk | 1 cup |
| 12:35 | turkey sub (tomato, lettuce, peppers, low-fat mayo) | 6" sub |
| | baby carrots | around 10 |
| | diet soda | 12 oz. can |
| 2:30 | apple slices with peanut butter | 1 medium |
| 6:00 | grilled chicken | 1 breast |
| | | 1/2 cup |

## Lose It! — HABIT TRACKER

Record your success with Add, Break and Bonus habits.

### WEEK 1 HABIT TRACKER

| ✓ Check if done | Day 1 | Day 2 | Day 3 | Day 4 | Day 5 | Day 6 | Day 7 | TOTALS |
|---|---|---|---|---|---|---|---|---|
| **ADD 5 HABITS** | | | | | | | | |
| 1. Eat a healthy breakfast | | | | ✓ | | ✓ | ✓ | 5 |
| 2. Eat vegetables and fruits | ✓ | ✓ | | | | ✓ | ✓ | 5 |
| 3. Eat whole grains | ✓ | ✓ | ✓ | | ✓ | | ✓ | 5 |
| 4. Eat healthy fats | ✓ | ✓ | ✓ | | | ✓ | ✓ | 6 |
| 5. Move! | ✓ | ✓ | ✓ | ✓ | ✓ | ✓ | ✓ | 5 |
| **BREAK 5 HABITS** | | ✓ | | | | | ✓ | 3 |
| 1. No TV while eating | | | | ✓ | | ✓ | ✓ | 6 |
| 2. No sugar | | ✓ | ✓ | ✓ | | ✓ | ✓ | |

## Lose It! — REVIEW

Re-examine how *Lose It!* went on the pages below.

| My start weight | 185 |
|---|---|
| Minus my weight today | 177 |
| = Equals my weight change | 8 |

**I FEEL:**
- ✓ Terrific
- ○ Good
- ○ So-so
- ○ Discouraged
- ○ Like giving up

**THE RESULTS FROM *LOSE IT!*:**
- ○ Far exceeded my expectations
- ✓ Were better than I expected
- ○ Met my expectations
- ○ Were not as good as I expected
- ○ Fell far short of my expectations

### ASSESSING YOUR HABIT TRACKER:

Days

| | 1 | 2 | 3 | 4 | 5 | 6 | 7 | 8 | 9 | 10 | 11 | 12 | 13 | 14 |
|---|---|---|---|---|---|---|---|---|---|---|---|---|---|---|
| 15 | | | | | | | | | | | | | | |
| 14 | | | | | | | | | | | | | | |

| WEEK 1 HABIT TRACKER | | | | | | | | |
|---|---|---|---|---|---|---|---|---|
| ✓ Check if done | Day 1 | Day 2 | Day 3 | Day 4 | Day 5 | Day 6 | Day 7 | TOTALS |
| **ADD 5 HABITS** | | | | | | | | |
| 1. Eat a healthy breakfast | | | | | | | | |
| 2. Eat vegetables and fruits | | | | | | | | |
| 3. Eat whole grains | | | | | | | | |
| 4. Eat healthy fats | | | | | | | | |
| 5. Move! | | | | | | | | |
| **BREAK 5 HABITS** | | | | | | | | |
| 1. No TV while eating | | | | | | | | |
| 2. No sugar | | | | | | | | |
| 3. No snacks | | | | | | | | |
| 4. Only moderate meat and dairy | | | | | | | | |
| 5. No eating at restaurants | | | | | | | | |
| **5 BONUS HABITS** | | | | | | | | |
| 1. Keep diet records | | | | | | | | |
| 2. Keep exercise/activity records | | | | | | | | |
| 3. Move more! | | | | | | | | |
| 4. Eat "real" food | | | | | | | | |
| 5. Write your daily goals | | | | | | | | |
| **Totals** | | | | | | | | |

**DIRECTIONS:**

1. At the end of each day, check off which Add, Break and Bonus habits you have completed.
2. At the end of the week, total the columns and the rows to see how you've progressed.

| WEEK 2 HABIT TRACKER | | | | | | | |
|---|---|---|---|---|---|---|---|
| Day 8 | Day 9 | Day 10 | Day 11 | Day 12 | Day 13 | Day 14 | TOTALS |
| **ADD 5 HABITS** | | | | | | | |
| | | | | | | | |
| | | | | | | | |
| | | | | | | | |
| | | | | | | | |
| | | | | | | | |
| **BREAK 5 HABITS** | | | | | | | |
| | | | | | | | |
| | | | | | | | |
| | | | | | | | |
| | | | | | | | |
| | | | | | | | |
| **5 BONUS HABITS** | | | | | | | |
| | | | | | | | |
| | | | | | | | |
| | | | | | | | |
| | | | | | | | |
| | | | | | | | |

# HABIT TRACKER

**REMINDER:**

Total the columns and rows of your Habit Tracker to see which habits you're having success with and which are a problem for you.

See pages 58-59 of *The Mayo Clinic Diet*.

| WEEK 1 HABIT T | | | |
|---|---|---|---|
| ✓ Check if done | Day 1 | Day 2 | Day |
| **ADD 5 HABITS** | | | |
| 1. Eat a healthy breakfast | ✓ | ✓ | |
| 2. Eat vegetables and fruits | ✓ | ✓ | ✓ |
| 3. Eat whole grains | ✓ | ✓ | ✓ |
| 4. Eat healthy fats | ✓ | ✓ | ✓ |
| 5. Move! | ✓ | | |
| **BREAK 5 HABITS** | | | |
| 1. No TV while eating | | | |
| 2. No sugar | | ✓ | ✓ |
| 3. No snacks | | ✓ | ✓ |
| 4. Only moderate meat and dairy | ✓ | ✓ | ✓ |
| 5. No eating at restaurants | ✓ | ✓ | ✓ |
| **5 BONUS HABITS** | | | |

The sample above demonstrates how to fill out your Habit Tracker.

**DAY 1**

**TODAY'S GOAL:**

**TODAY'S ACTIVITIES:**   🕐 Time

| | |
|---|---|
| | |
| | |
| **Total time (in minutes)** | |

**MY START WEIGHT:**

**WHAT I ATE TODAY:**

| 🕐 Time | Food item | Amount |
|---|---|---|
| | | |
| | | |
| | | |
| | | |
| | | |
| | | |
| | | |
| | | |
| | | |
| | | |
| | | |

**DAY 2**

**TODAY'S GOAL:**

**TODAY'S ACTIVITIES:**   🕐 Time

| | |
|---|---|
| | |
| | |
| | |
| Total time (in minutes) | |

**MOTIVATION TIP:**
Write down all the benefits of losing weight. Rank your top three reasons. Refer to the list frequently.

**WHAT I ATE TODAY:**

| 🕐 Time | Food item | Amount |
|---|---|---|
| | | |
| | | |
| | | |
| | | |
| | | |
| | | |
| | | |
| | | |
| | | |
| | | |
| | | |
| | | |
| | | |
| | | |

**DAY 3**

**TODAY'S GOAL:**

**TODAY'S ACTIVITIES:**                                    🕐 **Time**

| | |
|---|---|
| | |
| | |
| | |
| | |
| **Total time (in minutes)** | |

**MOTIVATION TIP:**
It takes time for the healthy new behaviors you're learning to become habits. Every step, every day, is important.

**WHAT I ATE TODAY:**

| 🕐 Time | Food item | Amount |
|---------|-----------|--------|
| | | |
| | | |
| | | |
| | | |
| | | |
| | | |
| | | |
| | | |
| | | |
| | | |
| | | |
| | | |
| | | |

**DAY 4**

**TODAY'S GOAL:**

**TODAY'S ACTIVITIES:** | Time

|  |  |
|  |  |
|  |  |
|  |  |
| Total time (in minutes) | |

**MOTIVATION TIP:**

Getting support from others is not a sign of weakness. If you feel that you need help, ask for it.

**WHAT I ATE TODAY:**

| Time | Food item | Amount |
|------|-----------|--------|
|      |           |        |
|      |           |        |
|      |           |        |
|      |           |        |
|      |           |        |
|      |           |        |
|      |           |        |
|      |           |        |
|      |           |        |
|      |           |        |
|      |           |        |
|      |           |        |

**DAY**
**5**

**TODAY'S GOAL:**

**TODAY'S ACTIVITIES:**   🕐 Time

| | | |
|---|---|---|
| | | |
| | | |
| | | |
| Total time (in minutes) | | |

**MOTIVATION TIP:**

Learning to say no to things that aren't essential gives you time for things you really want to do.

**WHAT I ATE TODAY:**

| 🕐 Time | Food item | Amount |
|---|---|---|
| | | |
| | | |
| | | |
| | | |
| | | |
| | | |
| | | |
| | | |
| | | |
| | | |
| | | |
| | | |

**DAY 6**

**TODAY'S GOAL:**

**TODAY'S ACTIVITIES:** 🕐 Time

| | |
|---|---|
| | |
| | |
| | |
| | |
| Total time (in minutes) | |

**MOTIVATION TIP:**
Check restaurant Web sites for menus. You can look for healthy options before you eat there.

**WHAT I ATE TODAY:**

| 🕐 Time | Food item | Amount |
|---|---|---|
| | | |
| | | |
| | | |
| | | |
| | | |
| | | |
| | | |
| | | |
| | | |
| | | |
| | | |

**TODAY'S GOAL:**

**TODAY'S ACTIVITIES:**  🕐 Time

| | |
|---|---|
| | |
| | |
| | |
| **Total time (in minutes)** | |

**MY WEIGHT TODAY:**

**WHAT I ATE TODAY:**

| 🕐 Time | Food item | Amount |
|---|---|---|
| | | |
| | | |
| | | |
| | | |
| | | |
| | | |
| | | |
| | | |
| | | |
| | | |

DAY
7

**TODAY'S GOAL:**

**TODAY'S ACTIVITIES:**     🕐 Time

| | |
|---|---|
| | |
| | |
| | |
| Total time (in minutes) | |

**DAY 8**

MOTIVATION TIP:

Change your exercise routine occasionally and do a variety of activities to avoid workout boredom.

**WHAT I ATE TODAY:**

| 🕐 Time | Food item | Amount |
|---|---|---|
| | | |
| | | |
| | | |
| | | |
| | | |
| | | |
| | | |
| | | |
| | | |

**DAY**
**9**

**TODAY'S GOAL:**

**TODAY'S ACTIVITIES:**    🕐 Time

| | |
|---|---|
| | |
| | |
| | |
| Total time (in minutes) | |

**MOTIVATION TIP:**
Don't think too far ahead. Look at what you can do today to make your program work for you.

**WHAT I ATE TODAY:**

| 🕐 Time | Food item | Amount |
|---|---|---|
| | | |
| | | |
| | | |
| | | |
| | | |
| | | |
| | | |
| | | |
| | | |
| | | |
| | | |
| | | |

**DAY 10**

**TODAY'S GOAL:**

| TODAY'S ACTIVITIES: | 🕐 Time |
|---|---|
|  |  |
|  |  |
|  |  |
|  |  |
| Total time (in minutes) |  |

**MOTIVATION TIP:**

Reward yourself with something that matters to you every time you reach a goal.

**WHAT I ATE TODAY:**

| 🕐 Time | Food item | Amount |
|---|---|---|
|  |  |  |
|  |  |  |
|  |  |  |
|  |  |  |
|  |  |  |
|  |  |  |
|  |  |  |
|  |  |  |
|  |  |  |
|  |  |  |
|  |  |  |

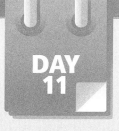

**DAY 11**

## TODAY'S GOAL:

## TODAY'S ACTIVITIES:                              🕐 Time

|  |  |  |
|--|--|--|
|  |  |  |
|  |  |  |
| Total time (in minutes) |  |  |

**MOTIVATION TIP:**
Choose exercises that you can do regardless of the weather, such as mall walking or indoor swimming.

## WHAT I ATE TODAY:

| 🕐 Time | Food item | Amount |
|---------|-----------|--------|
|  |  |  |
|  |  |  |
|  |  |  |
|  |  |  |
|  |  |  |
|  |  |  |
|  |  |  |
|  |  |  |
|  |  |  |
|  |  |  |

**DAY 12**

**TODAY'S GOAL:**

**TODAY'S ACTIVITIES:** 🕐 Time

|  |  |
|---|---|
|  |  |
|  |  |
|  |  |
| **Total time (in minutes)** |  |

**MOTIVATION TIP:**
Weight-loss goals may change over time. Review them periodically and make sure they're still realistic.

**WHAT I ATE TODAY:**

| 🕐 Time | Food item | Amount |
|---|---|---|
|  |  |  |
|  |  |  |
|  |  |  |
|  |  |  |
|  |  |  |
|  |  |  |
|  |  |  |
|  |  |  |
|  |  |  |
|  |  |  |

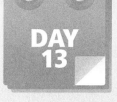

**DAY 13**

**TODAY'S GOAL:**

**TODAY'S ACTIVITIES:**                    🕐 Time

| | | |
|---|---|---|
| | | |
| | | |
| **Total time (in minutes)** | | |

**MOTIVATION TIP:**
Negative self-talk can produce anxiety. Be aware of what you say to yourself and try to make it more positive.

**WHAT I ATE TODAY:**

| 🕐 Time | Food item | Amount |
|---|---|---|
| | | |
| | | |
| | | |
| | | |
| | | |
| | | |
| | | |
| | | |
| | | |
| | | |

**DAY 14**

## TODAY'S GOAL:

## TODAY'S ACTIVITIES:
🕐 Time

| | |
|---|---|
| | |
| | |
| **Total time (in minutes)** | |

**MY WEIGHT TODAY:**

## WHAT I ATE TODAY:

| 🕐 Time | Food item | Amount |
|---------|-----------|--------|
| | | |
| | | |
| | | |
| | | |
| | | |
| | | |
| | | |
| | | |
| | | |
| | | |
| | | |

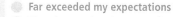

| My start weight | |
| --- | --- |
| Minus my weight today | |
| = Equals my weight change | |

**I FEEL:**
- Terrific
- Good
- So-so
- Discouraged
- Like giving up

**THE RESULTS FROM *LOSE IT!*:**
- Far exceeded my expectations
- Were better than I expected
- Met my expectations
- Were not as good as I expected
- Fell far short of my expectations

## ASSESSING YOUR HABIT TRACKER:

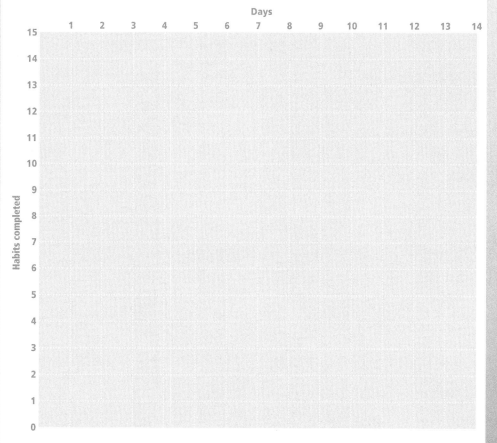

**DIRECTIONS:**

For each day of *Lose It!*, mark a dot on the graph to indicate the number of check marks you entered in your Habit Tracker. Then connect the dots to show the entire 14 days.

See a sample chart on the next page →

**NOTE:**

On some days you'll have fewer check marks than on other days — that's to be expected. But on most days, consider 10 check marks to be a reasonable mark of success. The days when you have more than 10 check marks are all the better!

## WHICH HABITS WERE STRENGTHS FOR YOU? CAN YOU LIST REASONS WHY YOU DID WELL?

LOSE IT!

# REVIEW

**HOW MOTIVATED ARE YOU TO TRANSITION INTO *LIVE IT!*?**
- Extremely
- Confident
- Somewhat
- Not very
- Not at all

See page 61 of *The Mayo Clinic Diet.*

## WHICH HABITS DID YOU FIND MOST CHALLENGING? WHY WERE THEY MORE DIFFICULT?

## CAN YOU SEE TRENDS ON YOUR HABIT TRACKER?
(for example, a strong start but then lost momentum or a difference between weekdays and weekends)

ASSESSING YOUR HABIT TRACKER:

## CAN YOU IDENTIFY STRATEGIES TO HELP YOU AVOID CHALLENGING OR DISRUPTIVE SITUATIONS?

The sample above shows how you can fill out your Habit Tracker assessment.

# Live It!

This section of *The Mayo Clinic Diet Journal* is designed to help you continue losing weight — now at a more sustainable 1 to 2 pounds a week — until you reach your goal weight, and then to maintain that weight as you *Live It!* for the rest of your life.

# How to plan *Live It!*

Start each week with the Planner, which can help organize your week and guide your food and exercise decisions.

**1** Use the Week At A Glance to create an overview of your meals, exercise and activity schedule, and events and special plans for the week ahead.

**2** The Meal Planner allows you to check how well a meal fits in your daily recommended servings goals. This is an optional feature that you may choose for one or two meals during the week.

**3** Add items to the Shopping List as you plan your daily menus. That will help you save time and money on your next shopping trip.

**1**

**Live It!**

WEEK 2 PLANNER · WEEK AT A GLANCE

| Day | Breakfast | Lunch | Dinner | Snack |
|---|---|---|---|---|
| EXAMPLE | cereal banana | spaghetti fruit salad | tuna wrap baby carrots | crackers and cheese |
| 1 | blueberry pancake milk | dilled pasta salad apple | rosemary chicken baked potato cauliflower | cherry tomatoes |
| 2 | toast & jam grapefruit | California burger pear | Greek salad crackers | baby carrots & dip |
| 3 | fruit yogurt parfait small muffin | turkey sandwich mixed greens with dressing | pasta primavera apple | celery & peanut butter |
| 4 | muffins pear halves | chicken wrap sliced tomato | beef kebabs potatoes pineapple ring | mixed berries |
| 5 | English muffin grapefruit | Southwestern salad pita bread | spaghetti with tomato sauce zucchini | peanuts |
| 6 | hard-boiled egg toast orange | pita bread with hummus cucumber & tomato salad | grilled fish brown rice Brussels sprouts | cherries |

| MAIN MEAL OR MEALS OF THE DAY | HOW MUCH |
|---|---|
| Dinner | |
| grilled chicken breast | 2 1/2 oz |
| baby potatoes | 3 |
| steamed broccoli | 2 cups |
| margarine | 1 tsp |
| pear | 1 small |

WEEK 2 PLANNER

## MEAL PLANNER

EASY AS 1, 2, 3:
This page allows you to check how well a meal meets your recommended servings goals.

❶ Write down what you're planning to eat for that meal for each

| Fresh produce | Whole grains | Meat & dairy |
|---|---|---|
| 10 large tomatoes | 8 oz. package spaghetti | salmon fillets |
| 2 red peppers | 1 loaf rye bread | chicken breasts |
| summer squash | 1 package English muffins | milk |
| zucchini | | yogurt |
| 1 bag baby carrots | bag of pita bread | |
| cherries | | |
| 3 grapefruit | | |

WEEK 2 PLANNER

## SHOPPING LIST

PLAN AHEAD:
Create your Shopping List the week before going to the grocery store. You'll have all the ingredients on hand or the time you all

# How to record *Live It!*

**1** Start each day by setting a realistic, achievable goal in the Daily Record.

**2** Record everything you eat, including amounts and the number of pyramid servings.

**3** Record how much time you spend doing exercise and being active. Activity should be moderately intense and sustained for five minutes or more.

**4** Following day 7, take time to assess your progress in the weekly Review.

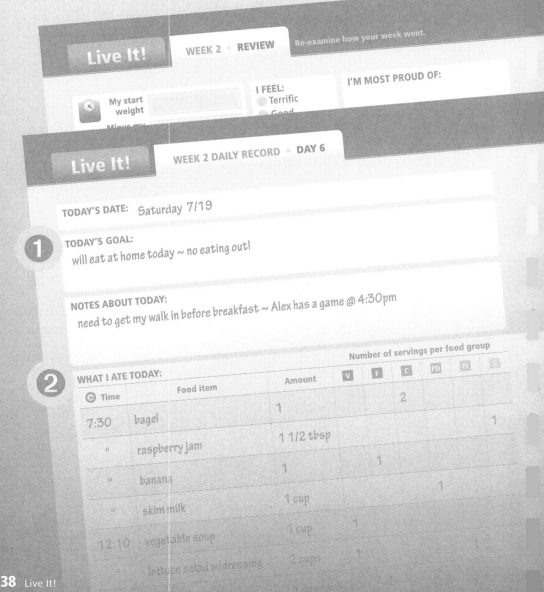

### Live It!    WEEK 2 • REVIEW    Re-examine how your week went.

My start weight

Minus my

**I FEEL:**
- Terrific
- Good

**I'M MOST PROUD OF:**

### Live It!    WEEK 2 DAILY RECORD • DAY 6

**TODAY'S DATE:** Saturday 7/19

**1**

**TODAY'S GOAL:**
will eat at home today ~ no eating out!

**NOTES ABOUT TODAY:**
need to get my walk in before breakfast ~ Alex has a game @ 4:30pm

**2 WHAT I ATE TODAY:**

| Time | Food item | Amount | V | F | C | PD | Fa | S |
|------|-----------|--------|---|---|---|----|----|----|
| 7:30 | bagel | 1 | | | 2 | | | |
| " | raspberry jam | 1 1/2 tbsp | | | | | | 1 |
| " | banana | 1 | | 1 | | | | |
| " | skim milk | 1 cup | | | | 1 | | |
| 12:10 | vegetable soup | 1 cup | 1 | | | | | |
| " | lettuce salad w/dressing | 2 cups | 1 | | | | 1 | |
| | yogurt w/cereal | 1 cup each | | | | | | |

*Number of servings per food group*

NEW FOOD I WOULD LIKE TO TRY:

WEEK 2

# DAY 6

| TODAY'S ACTIVITIES: | 🕐 Time |
|---|---|
| early morning walk | 30 minutes |
| mow the lawn | 45 minutes |
| walk to the ballgame | 15 minutes |
| | |
| Total time (in minutes) | 90 minutes |

③

**MOTIVATION TIP:** Different fruits provide different nutrients, so variety is vital to get all the health benefits. Use them for snacks and at every meal.

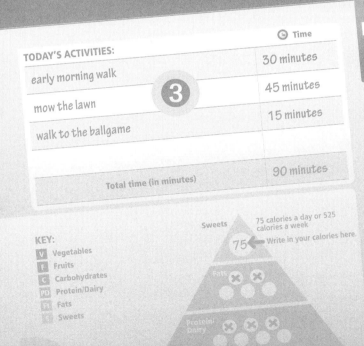

Sweets    75 calories a day or 525 calories a week

75 ← Write in your calories here.

KEY:
- **V** Vegetables
- **t** Fruits
- **C** Carbohydrates
- **PD** Protein/Dairy
- **R** Fats
- **S** Sweets

Fats

Protein/ Dairy

Carbohydrates

| Day | Breakfast | Lunch | Dinner | Snack |
|---|---|---|---|---|
| EXAMPLE | cereal banana | spaghetti fruit salad | tuna wrap baby carrots | crackers and cheese |
| 1 | | | | |
| 2 | | | | |
| 3 | | | | |
| 4 | | | | |
| 5 | | | | |
| 6 | | | | |
| 7 | | | | |

# WEEK AT A GLANCE

| Exercise and activities | Events and special plans |
|---|---|
| swim class @ 11am<br>walk to work | kids ballgame @ 6pm<br>note: supper will be on the go |
| | |
| | |
| | |
| | |
| | |
| | |
| | |

**USING THE PLANNER:**

Organize your plans for meals, activities and exercise in the coming week. Note upcoming events that may affect your weight program, such as travel, eating out, social occasions and vacations.

| MAIN MEAL OR MEALS OF THE DAY | HOW MUCH |
|---|---|
|  |  |

**EASY AS 1, 2, 3:**

This page allows you to check how well a meal meets your recommended servings goals.

1. Write down what you're planning to eat for this meal (or for the entire day).
2. Calculate the number of servings based on how much you're planning to eat.
3. Be sure to include the food items from your menu in your Shopping List.

## PYRAMID SERVINGS FOR THIS MEAL

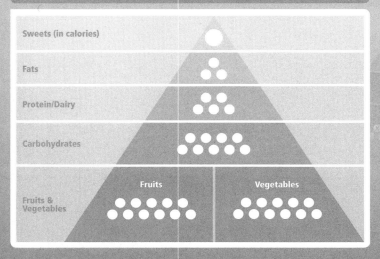

Sweets (in calories)

Fats

Protein/Dairy

Carbohydrates

Fruits &
Vegetables — Fruits — Vegetables

◄ Check off the number of servings on the pyramid at left.

**WEEK 1 PLANNER**

# MEAL PLANNER

| MAIN MEAL OR MEALS OF THE DAY | HOW MUCH |
|---|---|
| | |

EASY AS 1, 2, 3:

This page allows you to check how well a meal meets your recommended servings goals.

1. Write down what you're planning to eat for this meal (or for the entire day).
2. Calculate the number of servings based on how much you're planning to eat.
3. Be sure to include the food items from your menu in your Shopping List.

## PYRAMID SERVINGS FOR THIS MEAL

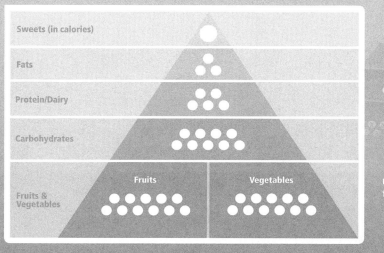

Sweets (in calories)

Fats

Protein/Dairy

Carbohydrates

Fruits & Vegetables

Fruits

Vegetables

75

◀ Check off the number of servings on the pyramid at left.

## MENU FOR THE DAY

### BREAKFAST

1 medium hard-boiled egg
1 slice whole-grain toast
1 tsp. trans-free margarine
*1 medium orange
Calorie-free beverage

| V | F | C | PD | Ft | S |
|---|---|---|----|----|---|
| 0 | 1 | 1 | 1 | 1 | 0 |

### LUNCH

Open-faced roast beef sandwich
*8 cherry tomatoes
*1 small apple
Calorie-free beverage

| V | F | C | PD | Ft | S |
|---|---|---|----|----|---|
| 1 | 1 | 1 | 1 | 0 | 0 |

### DINNER

1 serving Pasta with Marinara Sauce
   and Grilled Vegetables
¾ c. blueberries with ½ c. nondairy
   whipped topping
Calorie-free beverage

| V | F | C | PD | Ft | S |
|---|---|---|----|----|---|
| 3 | 1 | 2 | 0 | 2 | 0 |

### SNACK

1   c. fat-free, reduced-calorie yogurt

| V | F | C | PD | Ft | S |
|---|---|---|----|----|---|
| 0 | 0 | 0 | 1 | 0 | 0 |

*The serving size stated is the minimum
amount. Eat as much as you wish.

**QUICK TIP:**

The menu
on this page
demonstrates
how you can plan
your own daily
menus. Feel free
to include this
sample on one of
your days.

## DINNER RECIPE

## Pasta With Marinara Sauce and Grilled Vegetables

2   tbsp. olive oil
10  large fresh tomatoes, peeled
    and diced
1   tsp. salt
½   tsp. minced garlic
2   tbsp. chopped onion
1   tsp. dried basil
1   tsp. sugar
½   tsp. oregano
    Black pepper, to taste
2   red peppers, sliced into chunks
1   yellow summer squash, sliced
    lengthwise
1   zucchini, sliced lengthwise
1   sweet onion, sliced into ¼-inch
    rounds
1   8-oz. package of whole-wheat
    spaghetti

■  Heat oil in a heavy skillet.
   Add tomatoes, salt, garlic,
   onions, basil, sugar, oregano
   and black pepper. Cook slowly,
   uncovered, for 30 minutes or
   until sauce is thickened.

■  Brush peppers, squash, zucchini
   and onion with oil. Place
   under broiler and cook, turning
   frequently until browned and
   tender. Remove to bowl.

■  Cook spaghetti until al dente.
   Drain well and portion onto
   plates. Cover with equal
   amounts of sauce. Top with
   equal amounts of vegetables.
   Serve immediately.

**WEEK 1 PLANNER**

# SHOPPING LIST

| Fresh produce | Whole grains | Meat & dairy |
|---|---|---|
| | | |

| Frozen goods | Canned goods | Miscellaneous |
|---|---|---|
| | | |

**QUICK TIP:**

Create your shopping list for the week before going to the grocery store. You'll have all the ingredients on hand at the time you prepare a meal.

| Fresh produce | Whole grain |
|---|---|
| 10 large tomatoes | 8 oz package spaghetti |
| 2 red peppers | 1 loaf rye bre |
| summer squash | 1 package en muffins |
| zucchini | |
| 1 bag baby carrots | bag of pita |
| cherries | |
| 3 grapefruit | |

Add to your Shopping List as you plan your menus for the week.

**TODAY'S DATE:**

**TODAY'S GOAL:**

**NOTES ABOUT TODAY:**

**WHAT I ATE TODAY:** | | | | | Number of servings per food group | | | | |

| ⏱ Time | Food item | Amount | V | F | C | PD | Ft | S |
|---------|-----------|--------|---|---|---|----|----|----|
|  |  |  |  |  |  |  |  |  |
|  |  |  |  |  |  |  |  |  |
|  |  |  |  |  |  |  |  |  |
|  |  |  |  |  |  |  |  |  |
|  |  |  |  |  |  |  |  |  |
|  |  |  |  |  |  |  |  |  |
|  |  |  |  |  |  |  |  |  |
|  |  |  |  |  |  |  |  |  |
|  |  |  |  |  |  |  |  |  |
|  |  |  |  |  |  |  |  |  |

## TODAY'S ACTIVITIES:

🕐 Time

|  |  |
|--|--|
|  |  |
|  |  |
|  |  |
| **Total time (in minutes)** |  |

**MOTIVATION TIP:**
Don't worry too much about recording the exact number of servings of vegetables and fruits. You can eat, within reason, unlimited amounts from these two food groups.

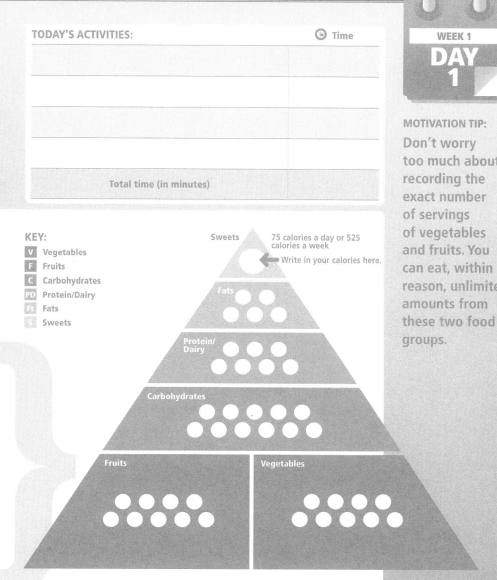

**KEY:**

- **V** Vegetables
- **F** Fruits
- **C** Carbohydrates
- **PD** Protein/Dairy
- **Ft** Fats
- **S** Sweets

Sweets — 75 calories a day or 525 calories a week
← Write in your calories here.

Fats

Protein/Dairy

Carbohydrates

Fruits

Vegetables

## WHAT I ATE TODAY FROM THE PYRAMID:

Check off the circles in the food group servings above as you record food and beverage items in the table at left. For sweets, give your best estimate of the total number of calories for the day.

**TODAY'S DATE:**

**TODAY'S GOAL:**

**NOTES ABOUT TODAY:**

**WHAT I ATE TODAY:**

Number of servings per food group

| Time | Food item | Amount | V | F | C | PD | Ft | S |
|------|-----------|--------|---|---|---|----|----|----|
|      |           |        |   |   |   |    |    |   |
|      |           |        |   |   |   |    |    |   |
|      |           |        |   |   |   |    |    |   |
|      |           |        |   |   |   |    |    |   |
|      |           |        |   |   |   |    |    |   |
|      |           |        |   |   |   |    |    |   |
|      |           |        |   |   |   |    |    |   |
|      |           |        |   |   |   |    |    |   |
|      |           |        |   |   |   |    |    |   |
|      |           |        |   |   |   |    |    |   |

**TODAY'S ACTIVITIES:**                                  🕐 Time

| | |
|---|---|
| | |
| | |
| | |
| **Total time (in minutes)** | |

**MOTIVATION TIP:**

A common mistake is to start off exercising too much and too hard. If your body isn't used to this exertion, your muscles may feel stiff and sore, causing you to exercise less or skip it altogether.

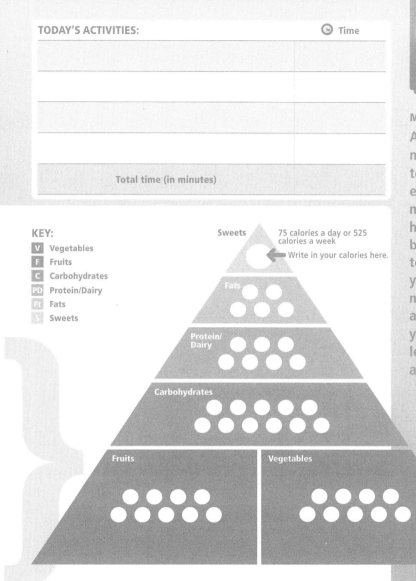

**KEY:**
- V   Vegetables
- F   Fruits
- C   Carbohydrates
- PD  Protein/Dairy
- Ft  Fats
- S   Sweets

Sweets
75 calories a day or 525 calories a week
Write in your calories here.

Fats

Protein/Dairy

Carbohydrates

Fruits

Vegetables

**WHAT I ATE TODAY FROM THE PYRAMID:**
Check off the circles in the food group servings above as you record food and beverage items in the table at left. For sweets, give your best estimate of the total number of calories for the day.

**TODAY'S DATE:**

**TODAY'S GOAL:**

**NOTES ABOUT TODAY:**

**WHAT I ATE TODAY:**

Number of servings per food group

| 🕐 Time | Food item | Amount | V | F | C | PD | Ft | S |
|---------|-----------|--------|---|---|---|----|----|---|
|  |  |  |  |  |  |  |  |  |
|  |  |  |  |  |  |  |  |  |
|  |  |  |  |  |  |  |  |  |
|  |  |  |  |  |  |  |  |  |
|  |  |  |  |  |  |  |  |  |
|  |  |  |  |  |  |  |  |  |
|  |  |  |  |  |  |  |  |  |
|  |  |  |  |  |  |  |  |  |
|  |  |  |  |  |  |  |  |  |
|  |  |  |  |  |  |  |  |  |
|  |  |  |  |  |  |  |  |  |

**TODAY'S ACTIVITIES:**                                    ⏱ Time

_____

_____

_____

_____

| **Total time (in minutes)** |

**MOTIVATION TIP:**

Friends — even spouses — may sometimes feel intimidated by your efforts to lose weight. It's up to you to let them know how important their support is to you.

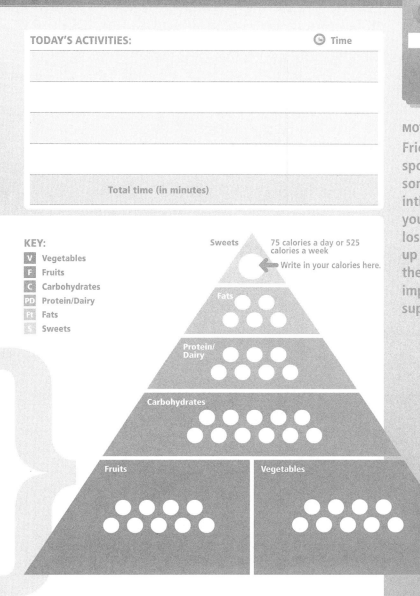

**KEY:**

| V | Vegetables |
| F | Fruits |
| C | Carbohydrates |
| PD | Protein/Dairy |
| Ft | Fats |
| S | Sweets |

Sweets — 75 calories a day or 525 calories a week
→ Write in your calories here.

Fats

Protein/Dairy

Carbohydrates

Fruits

Vegetables

**WHAT I ATE TODAY FROM THE PYRAMID:**

Check off the circles in the food group servings above as you record food and beverage items in the table at left. For sweets, give your best estimate of the total number of calories for the day.

**TODAY'S DATE:**

**TODAY'S GOAL:**

**NOTES ABOUT TODAY:**

**WHAT I ATE TODAY:**

**Number of servings per food group**

| Time | Food item | Amount | V | F | C | PD | Ft | S |
|------|-----------|--------|---|---|---|----|----|---|
|      |           |        |   |   |   |    |    |   |
|      |           |        |   |   |   |    |    |   |
|      |           |        |   |   |   |    |    |   |
|      |           |        |   |   |   |    |    |   |
|      |           |        |   |   |   |    |    |   |
|      |           |        |   |   |   |    |    |   |
|      |           |        |   |   |   |    |    |   |
|      |           |        |   |   |   |    |    |   |
|      |           |        |   |   |   |    |    |   |
|      |           |        |   |   |   |    |    |   |
|      |           |        |   |   |   |    |    |   |
|      |           |        |   |   |   |    |    |   |

**TODAY'S ACTIVITIES:**　🕐 **Time**

| | |
|---|---|
| | |
| | |
| | |
| | |
| **Total time (in minutes)** | |

**MOTIVATION TIP:**
When you know you'll be eating out (and eating extra calories), try to increase the amount of exercise you do on that day.

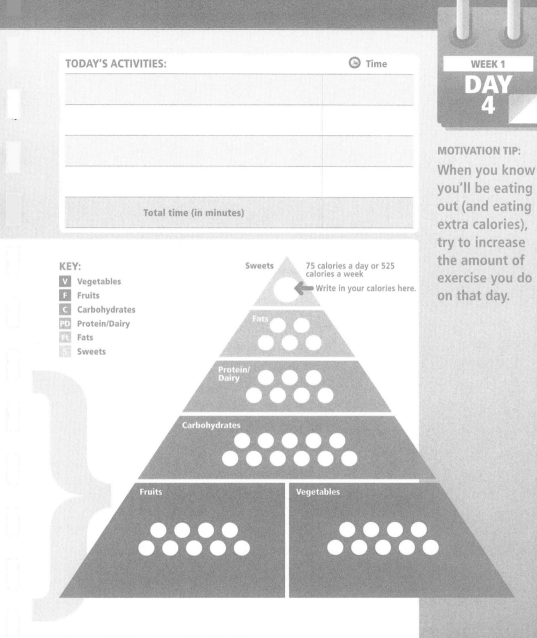

**KEY:**
- V Vegetables
- F Fruits
- C Carbohydrates
- PD Protein/Dairy
- Ft Fats
- S Sweets

Sweets

75 calories a day or 525 calories a week
← Write in your calories here.

Fats

Protein/Dairy

Carbohydrates

Fruits

Vegetables

**WHAT I ATE TODAY FROM THE PYRAMID:**
Check off the circles in the food group servings above as you record food and beverage items in the table at left. For sweets, give your best estimate of the total number of calories for the day.

**TODAY'S DATE:**

**TODAY'S GOAL:**

**NOTES ABOUT TODAY:**

**WHAT I ATE TODAY:**

Number of servings per food group

| Time | Food item | Amount | V | F | C | PD | Pt | S |
|---|---|---|---|---|---|---|---|---|
|  |  |  |  |  |  |  |  |  |
|  |  |  |  |  |  |  |  |  |
|  |  |  |  |  |  |  |  |  |
|  |  |  |  |  |  |  |  |  |
|  |  |  |  |  |  |  |  |  |
|  |  |  |  |  |  |  |  |  |
|  |  |  |  |  |  |  |  |  |
|  |  |  |  |  |  |  |  |  |
|  |  |  |  |  |  |  |  |  |
|  |  |  |  |  |  |  |  |  |
|  |  |  |  |  |  |  |  |  |

**TODAY'S ACTIVITIES:** 🕐 **Time**

| | |
|---|---|
| | |
| | |
| | |
| | |
| **Total time (in minutes)** | |

**MOTIVATION TIP:**
Choose activities that fit your personality. If you prefer solitude, consider walking or jogging. If group activities appeal to you, consider an aerobics class or golf league.

**KEY:**
- **V** Vegetables
- **F** Fruits
- **C** Carbohydrates
- **PD** Protein/Dairy
- **Ft** Fats
- **S** Sweets

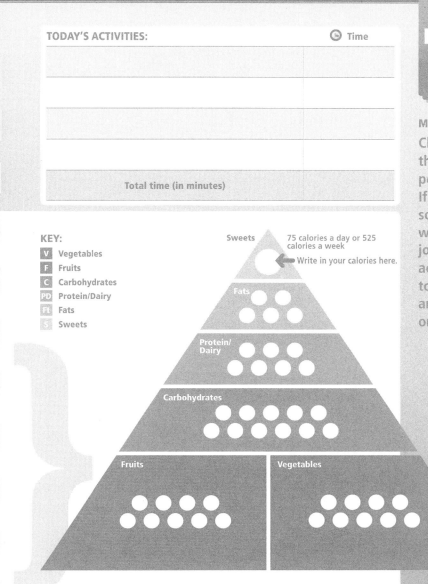

Sweets — 75 calories a day or 525 calories a week
← Write in your calories here.

Fats

Protein/Dairy

Carbohydrates

Fruits

Vegetables

**WHAT I ATE TODAY FROM THE PYRAMID:**
Check off the circles in the food group servings above as you record food and beverage items in the table at left. For sweets, give your best estimate of the total number of calories for the day.

**TODAY'S DATE:**

**TODAY'S GOAL:**

**NOTES ABOUT TODAY:**

**WHAT I ATE TODAY:**                                    Number of servings per food group

| 🕐 Time | Food item | Amount | V | F | C | PD | Ft | S |
|---------|-----------|--------|---|---|---|----|----|---|
|  |  |  |  |  |  |  |  |  |
|  |  |  |  |  |  |  |  |  |
|  |  |  |  |  |  |  |  |  |
|  |  |  |  |  |  |  |  |  |
|  |  |  |  |  |  |  |  |  |
|  |  |  |  |  |  |  |  |  |
|  |  |  |  |  |  |  |  |  |
|  |  |  |  |  |  |  |  |  |
|  |  |  |  |  |  |  |  |  |
|  |  |  |  |  |  |  |  |  |
|  |  |  |  |  |  |  |  |  |
|  |  |  |  |  |  |  |  |  |

**TODAY'S ACTIVITIES:**  Time

Total time (in minutes)

**MOTIVATION TIP:**
Learn to recognize true hunger and ignore cravings. If you ate just a couple of hours ago and your stomach isn't rumbling, give the craving time to pass before you reach for snack food.

**KEY:**

V Vegetables
F Fruits
C Carbohydrates
PD Protein/Dairy
Ft Fats
S Sweets

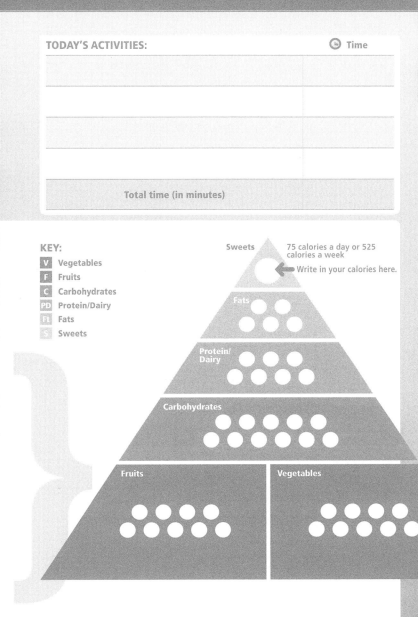

Sweets — 75 calories a day or 525 calories a week

Write in your calories here.

Fats

Protein/Dairy

Carbohydrates

Fruits

Vegetables

**WHAT I ATE TODAY FROM THE PYRAMID:**
Check off the circles in the food group servings above as you record food and beverage items in the table at left. For sweets, give your best estimate of the total number of calories for the day.

**TODAY'S DATE:**

**TODAY'S GOAL:**

**NOTES ABOUT TODAY:**
It's weigh-in day ~ record my weight in the weekly Review and the Weight Record.

**WHAT I ATE TODAY:**

Number of servings per food group

| ⏰ Time | Food item | Amount | V | F | C | PD | Pt | S |
|---------|-----------|--------|---|---|---|----|----|---|
| | | | | | | | | |
| | | | | | | | | |
| | | | | | | | | |
| | | | | | | | | |
| | | | | | | | | |
| | | | | | | | | |
| | | | | | | | | |
| | | | | | | | | |
| | | | | | | | | |
| | | | | | | | | |
| | | | | | | | | |
| | | | | | | | | |

## TODAY'S ACTIVITIES:

🕐 Time

|  |  |
|---|---|
|  |  |
|  |  |
|  |  |
| **Total time (in minutes)** |  |

WEEK 1

**DAY 7**

REMINDER:

Record your weight for today in the weekly Review and the Weight Record.

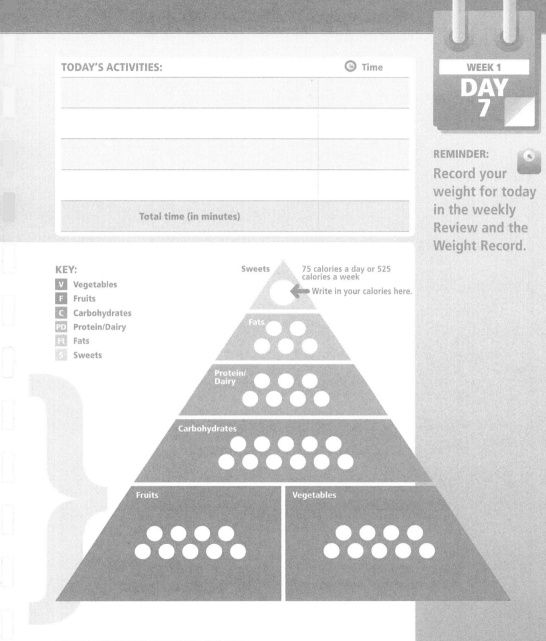

**KEY:**
- **V** Vegetables
- **F** Fruits
- **C** Carbohydrates
- **PD** Protein/Dairy
- **Ft** Fats
- **S** Sweets

Sweets — 75 calories a day or 525 calories a week

Write in your calories here.

Fats

Protein/Dairy

Carbohydrates

Fruits

Vegetables

## WHAT I ATE TODAY FROM THE PYRAMID:

Check off the circles in the food group servings above as you record food and beverage items in the table at left. For sweets, give your best estimate of the total number of calories for the day.

| My start weight | |
| Minus my weight today | |
| = Equals my weight change | |

**I FEEL:**
- Terrific
- Good
- So-so
- Discouraged
- Like giving up

**I'M MOST PROUD OF:**

**WHAT WORKED WELL:**

**WHAT DIDN'T WORK AS WELL:**

## DID I REACH MY SERVINGS GOALS FOR THIS WEEK?

| Food group | Daily servings | Day 1 | Day 2 | Day 3 | Day 4 | Day 5 | Day 6 | Day 7 |
|---|---|---|---|---|---|---|---|---|
| Vegetables | | ○ | ○ | ○ | ○ | ○ | ○ | ○ |
| Fruits | | ○ | ○ | ○ | ○ | ○ | ○ | ○ |
| Carbohydrates | | ○ | ○ | ○ | ○ | ○ | ○ | ○ |
| Protein/Dairy | | ○ | ○ | ○ | ○ | ○ | ○ | ○ |
| Fats | | ○ | ○ | ○ | ○ | ○ | ○ | ○ |
| Sweets | | ○ | ○ | ○ | ○ | ○ | ○ | ○ |

**DIRECTIONS:**
1. Write your daily serving goals for each food group in the table above.
2. Compare the serving totals that you recorded for each day of the past week with your goals.
3. Check off the circles in the table above if your serving totals have met your goals.

**NEW FOOD I WOULD LIKE TO TRY:**

**NEW WAYS TO ADD ACTIVITY TO MY DAY:**

**REMINDER:**
Calculate your weight change in this Review and record it in the Weight Record.

**HOW MANY STEPS A DAY DID I TAKE (IF I USED A PEDOMETER)?**

| Day 1 | Day 2 | Day 3 | Day 4 | Day 5 | Day 6 | Day 7 |
|-------|-------|-------|-------|-------|-------|-------|
|       |       |       |       |       |       |       |

**HOW MANY MINUTES A DAY WAS I ACTIVE?**

Days

| | 1 | 2 | 3 | 4 | 5 | 6 | 7 |

90
75
60
45
30
15
0

Minutes

**DIRECTIONS:**

1. Add a dot for your total minutes of activity for each day of last week.
2. Connect each dot on the chart with a line.

See a sample chart to the right. →

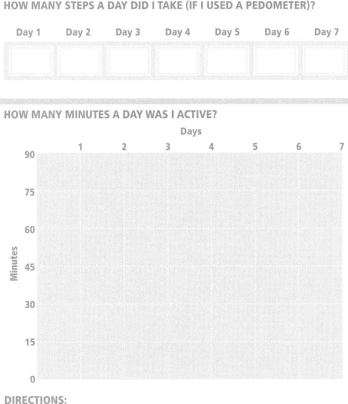

**DID I REACH MY SERVINGS GOALS FOR THIS W**

| Food group | Daily servings | Day 1 | Da |
|------------|----------------|-------|-----|
| Vegetables | 4+ | ✓ | |
| Fruits | 3+ | | ✓ |
| Carbohydrates | 4 | ✓ | ✓ |
| Protein/Dairy | 3 | ✓ | ✓ |
| | 3 | | ✓ |

The samples above show how you can fill out your servings goals table and your activity chart for your weekly Review.

| Day | Breakfast | Lunch | Dinner | Snack |
|---|---|---|---|---|
| EXAMPLE | cereal banana | spaghetti fruit salad | tuna wrap baby carrots | crackers and cheese |
| 1 | | | | |
| 2 | | | | |
| 3 | | | | |
| 4 | | | | |
| 5 | | | | |
| 6 | | | | |
| 7 | | | | |

| Exercise and activities | Events and special plans |
|---|---|
| swim class @ 11am<br>walk to work | kids ballgame @ 6pm<br>note: supper will be on the go |
| | |
| | |
| | |
| | |
| | |
| | |
| | |

# WEEK AT A GLANCE

**USING THE PLANNER:**

Organize your plans for meals, activities and exercise in the coming week. Note upcoming events that may affect your weight program, such as travel, eating out, social occasions and vacations.

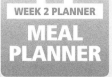

| MAIN MEAL OR MEALS OF THE DAY | HOW MUCH |
|---|---|
| | |

**EASY AS 1, 2, 3:**

This page allows you to check how well a meal meets your recommended servings goals.

1. Write down what you're planning to eat for this meal (or for the entire day).
2. Calculate the number of servings based on how much you're planning to eat.
3. Be sure to include the food items from your menu in your Shopping List.

## PYRAMID SERVINGS FOR THIS MEAL

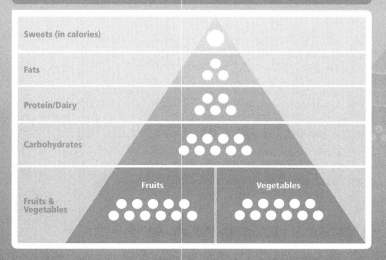

Sweets (in calories)

Fats

Protein/Dairy

Carbohydrates

Fruits

Vegetables

Fruits & Vegetables

◄ Check off the number of servings on the pyramid at left.

## WEEK 2 PLANNER
# MEAL PLANNER

| MAIN MEAL OR MEALS OF THE DAY | HOW MUCH |
|---|---|
|  |  |

**EASY AS 1, 2, 3:**

This page allows you to check how well a meal meets your recommended servings goals.

1. Write down what you're planning to eat for this meal (or for the entire day).
2. Calculate the number of servings based on how much you're planning to eat.
3. Be sure to include the food items from your menu in your Shopping List.

## PYRAMID SERVINGS FOR THIS MEAL

Sweets (in calories)

Fats

Protein/Dairy

Carbohydrates

Fruits & Vegetables — Fruits — Vegetables

75

◄ Check off the number of servings on the pyramid at left.

## MENU FOR THE DAY

### BREAKFAST
1 pancake (4-inch diameter)
*¾ c. blueberries or other berries
1 tsp. trans-free margarine
1½ tbsp. syrup
1 c. skim milk
Calorie-free beverage

| V | F | C | PD | Ft | S |
|---|---|---|----|----|---|
| 0 | 1 | 1 | 1  | 1  | 0 |

### LUNCH
1 serving Dilled Pasta Salad With
    Spring Vegetables
*1 small apple
Calorie-free beverage

| V | F | C | PD | Ft | S |
|---|---|---|----|----|---|
| 1 | 1 | 2 | 0  | 1  | 0 |

### DINNER
1 serving Rosemary Chicken
⅓ c. brown rice mixed with ½ cup
    chopped green onion
*1½ c. green beans
*1 medium orange
Calorie-free beverage

| V | F | C | PD | Ft | S |
|---|---|---|----|----|---|
| 3 | 1 | 1 | 2  | 1  | 0 |

### SNACK
*1 serving favorite fruit

| V | F | C | PD | Ft | S |
|---|---|---|----|----|---|
| 0 | 1 | 0 | 0  | 0  | 0 |

*The serving size stated is the minimum
amount. Eat as much as you wish.

QUICK TIP:

**The menu on this page demonstrates how you can plan your own daily menus. Feel free to include this sample on one of your days.**

## LUNCH RECIPE

### Dilled Pasta Salad With Spring Vegetables

3   c. shell pasta (medium-sized)
8   asparagus spears, cut into ½-inch pieces
1   c. halved cherry tomatoes
1   c. sliced green peppers
½   c. chopped green onions

**FOR THE DRESSING:**
¼   c. olive oil
2   tbsp. lemon juice
2   tbsp. rice or white wine vinegar
2   tsp. dill weed
Cracked black pepper, to taste

■ Cook and drain pasta. Rinse in cold water. Put into a bowl.

■ In a saucepan, cover asparagus with water. Cook until tender-crisp, 3 to 5 minutes. Drain and rinse with cold water. Add asparagus, tomatoes, green peppers and onions to pasta.

■ In a small bowl, whisk together the ingredients for the dressing. Pour dressing over the pasta and vegetables. Toss to coat. Cover, refrigerate and serve.

## DINNER RECIPE

### Rosemary Chicken

■ Brush a 5-ounce boneless, skinless chicken breast with 1 teaspoon each of olive oil, lemon juice and rosemary. Grill or bake.

| Fresh produce | Whole grains | Meat & dairy |
| --- | --- | --- |
| | | |

| Frozen goods | Canned goods | Miscellaneous |
| --- | --- | --- |
| | | |

WEEK 2 PLANNER

# SHOPPING LIST

QUICK TIP:

Create your shopping list for the week before going to the grocery store. You'll have all the ingredients on hand at the time you prepare a meal.

| Fresh produce | Whole grains |
| --- | --- |
| 10 large tomatoes | 8 oz package spaghetti |
| 2 red peppers | 1 loaf rye bread |
| summer squash | 1 package eng muffins |
| zucchini | bag of pita |
| 1 bag baby carrots | |
| cherries | |
| 3 grapefruit | |

Add to your Shopping List as you plan your menus for the week.

**TODAY'S DATE:**

**TODAY'S GOAL:**

**NOTES ABOUT TODAY:**

**WHAT I ATE TODAY:**

Number of servings per food group

| Time | Food item | Amount | V | F | C | PD | Ft | S |
|------|-----------|--------|---|---|---|----|----|---|
|      |           |        |   |   |   |    |    |   |
|      |           |        |   |   |   |    |    |   |
|      |           |        |   |   |   |    |    |   |
|      |           |        |   |   |   |    |    |   |
|      |           |        |   |   |   |    |    |   |
|      |           |        |   |   |   |    |    |   |
|      |           |        |   |   |   |    |    |   |
|      |           |        |   |   |   |    |    |   |
|      |           |        |   |   |   |    |    |   |
|      |           |        |   |   |   |    |    |   |
|      |           |        |   |   |   |    |    |   |
|      |           |        |   |   |   |    |    |   |

**TODAY'S ACTIVITIES:**

🕐 **Time**

| | |
|---|---|
| | |
| | |
| | |
| **Total time (in minutes)** | |

**MOTIVATION TIP:**
Increase your chances of sticking to your walking program by getting a walking buddy. A companion can help keep you motivated and make you feel safer.

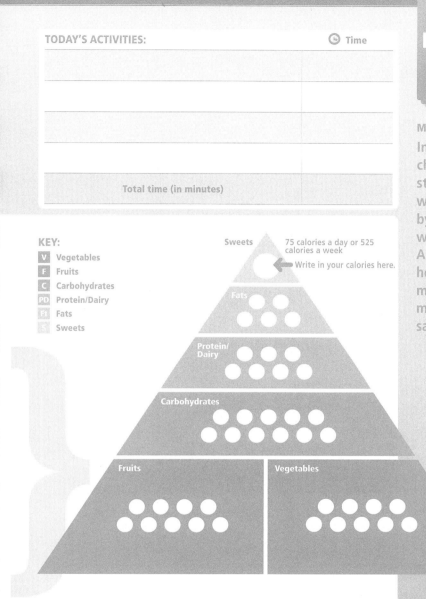

**KEY:**
- **V** Vegetables
- **F** Fruits
- **C** Carbohydrates
- **PD** Protein/Dairy
- **F** Fats
- **S** Sweets

**Sweets** — 75 calories a day or 525 calories a week
← Write in your calories here.

Fats

Protein/Dairy

Carbohydrates

Fruits

Vegetables

**WHAT I ATE TODAY FROM THE PYRAMID:**
Check off the circles in the food group servings above as you record food and beverage items in the table at left. For sweets, give your best estimate of the total number of calories for the day.

**TODAY'S DATE:**

**TODAY'S GOAL:**

**NOTES ABOUT TODAY:**

**WHAT I ATE TODAY:**

Number of servings per food group

| ⏱ Time | Food item | Amount | V | F | C | PD | Ft | S |
|--------|-----------|--------|---|---|---|----|----|---|
|        |           |        |   |   |   |    |    |   |
|        |           |        |   |   |   |    |    |   |
|        |           |        |   |   |   |    |    |   |
|        |           |        |   |   |   |    |    |   |
|        |           |        |   |   |   |    |    |   |
|        |           |        |   |   |   |    |    |   |
|        |           |        |   |   |   |    |    |   |
|        |           |        |   |   |   |    |    |   |
|        |           |        |   |   |   |    |    |   |
|        |           |        |   |   |   |    |    |   |
|        |           |        |   |   |   |    |    |   |
|        |           |        |   |   |   |    |    |   |

**TODAY'S ACTIVITIES:**

🕐 **Time**

**Total time (in minutes)**

**MOTIVATION TIP:**
When you feel lonely, do you turn to food for comfort? When you're with friends, do you tend to overeat? Make a list of unhealthy behaviors and think of ways to change those behaviors.

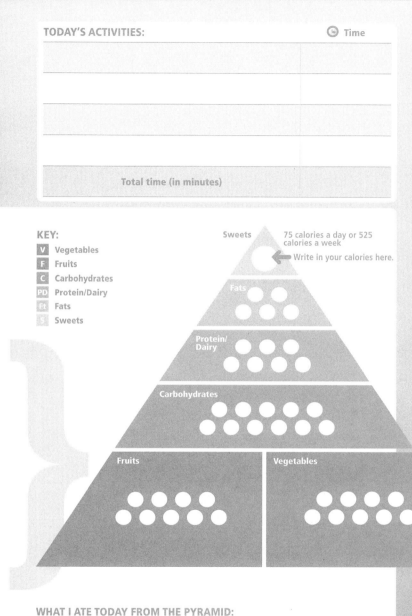

**KEY:**
- **V** Vegetables
- **F** Fruits
- **C** Carbohydrates
- **PD** Protein/Dairy
- **Ft** Fats
- **S** Sweets

Sweets

75 calories a day or 525 calories a week
← Write in your calories here.

Fats

Protein/Dairy

Carbohydrates

Fruits

Vegetables

**WHAT I ATE TODAY FROM THE PYRAMID:**
Check off the circles in the food group servings above as you record food and beverage items in the table at left. For sweets, give your best estimate of the total number of calories for the day.

**TODAY'S DATE:**

**TODAY'S GOAL:**

**NOTES ABOUT TODAY:**

**WHAT I ATE TODAY:**                                    Number of servings per food group

| ⏱ Time | Food item | Amount | V | F | C | PD | Ft | S |
|--------|-----------|--------|---|---|---|----|----|----|
|        |           |        |   |   |   |    |    |   |
|        |           |        |   |   |   |    |    |   |
|        |           |        |   |   |   |    |    |   |
|        |           |        |   |   |   |    |    |   |
|        |           |        |   |   |   |    |    |   |
|        |           |        |   |   |   |    |    |   |
|        |           |        |   |   |   |    |    |   |
|        |           |        |   |   |   |    |    |   |
|        |           |        |   |   |   |    |    |   |

**TODAY'S ACTIVITIES:**

🕐 Time

Total time (in minutes)

**MOTIVATION TIP:**
Keep foods that you crave out of the house or, at least, out of your sight. If you feel you must have a package of chocolate chips in the house, tuck them away in the back of a cupboard.

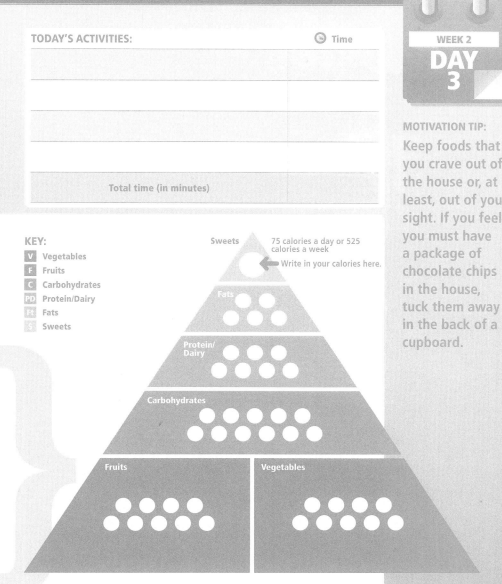

**KEY:**
- V Vegetables
- F Fruits
- C Carbohydrates
- PD Protein/Dairy
- Ft Fats
- S Sweets

Sweets

75 calories a day or 525 calories a week

Write in your calories here.

Fats

Protein/Dairy

Carbohydrates

Fruits

Vegetables

**WHAT I ATE TODAY FROM THE PYRAMID:**
Check off the circles in the food group servings above as you record food and beverage items in the table at left. For sweets, give your best estimate of the total number of calories for the day.

**TODAY'S DATE:**

**TODAY'S GOAL:**

**NOTES ABOUT TODAY:**

**WHAT I ATE TODAY:**                                    Number of servings per food group

| ⏰ Time | Food item | Amount | V | F | C | PD | Ft | S |
|---------|-----------|--------|---|---|---|----|----|----|
|  |  |  |  |  |  |  |  |  |
|  |  |  |  |  |  |  |  |  |
|  |  |  |  |  |  |  |  |  |
|  |  |  |  |  |  |  |  |  |
|  |  |  |  |  |  |  |  |  |
|  |  |  |  |  |  |  |  |  |
|  |  |  |  |  |  |  |  |  |
|  |  |  |  |  |  |  |  |  |
|  |  |  |  |  |  |  |  |  |
|  |  |  |  |  |  |  |  |  |
|  |  |  |  |  |  |  |  |  |
|  |  |  |  |  |  |  |  |  |

**TODAY'S ACTIVITIES:**                                    ⏱ Time

|  |  |
|---|---|
|  |  |
|  |  |
|  |  |
|  |  |
| **Total time (in minutes)** |  |

**MOTIVATION TIP:**

Try out a new activity that you've always wanted to do. Base your decision on personal appeal and not necessarily on what you think will help you lose weight.

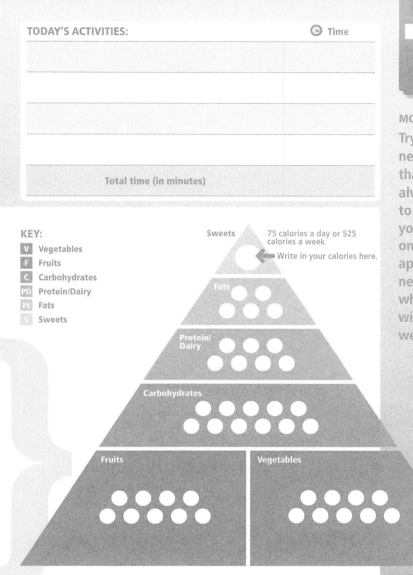

**KEY:**

- **V** Vegetables
- **F** Fruits
- **C** Carbohydrates
- **PD** Protein/Dairy
- **Ft** Fats
- **S** Sweets

Sweets — 75 calories a day or 525 calories a week
← Write in your calories here.

**WHAT I ATE TODAY FROM THE PYRAMID:**
Check off the circles in the food group servings above as you record food and beverage items in the table at left. For sweets, give your best estimate of the total number of calories for the day.

**TODAY'S DATE:**

**TODAY'S GOAL:**

**NOTES ABOUT TODAY:**

**WHAT I ATE TODAY:**

Number of servings per food group

| 🕐 Time | Food item | Amount | V | F | C | PD | Ft | S |
|---------|-----------|--------|---|---|---|----|----|---|
|  |  |  |  |  |  |  |  |  |
|  |  |  |  |  |  |  |  |  |
|  |  |  |  |  |  |  |  |  |
|  |  |  |  |  |  |  |  |  |
|  |  |  |  |  |  |  |  |  |
|  |  |  |  |  |  |  |  |  |
|  |  |  |  |  |  |  |  |  |
|  |  |  |  |  |  |  |  |  |
|  |  |  |  |  |  |  |  |  |
|  |  |  |  |  |  |  |  |  |
|  |  |  |  |  |  |  |  |  |
|  |  |  |  |  |  |  |  |  |
|  |  |  |  |  |  |  |  |  |

**TODAY'S ACTIVITIES:**

🕐 Time

Total time (in minutes)

**MOTIVATION TIP:**

Look for ways to make a favorite recipe more nutritious. This might include reducing the amount of sugar you add, using fat-free products and substituting legumes for meat.

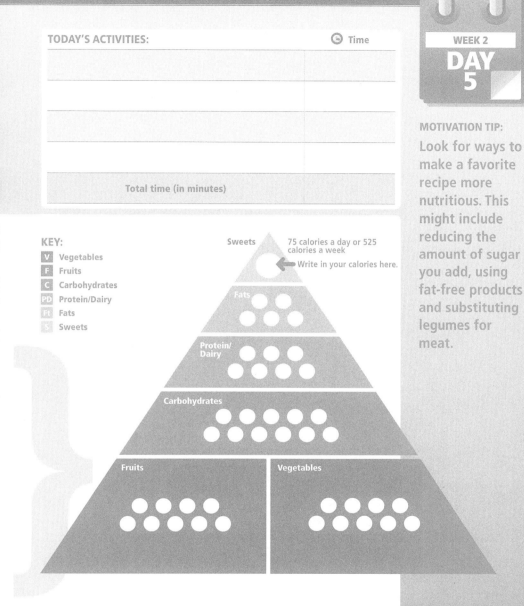

**KEY:**

**V** Vegetables
**F** Fruits
**C** Carbohydrates
**PD** Protein/Dairy
**Ft** Fats
**S** Sweets

Sweets — 75 calories a day or 525 calories a week

Write in your calories here.

Fats

Protein/Dairy

Carbohydrates

Fruits

Vegetables

**WHAT I ATE TODAY FROM THE PYRAMID:**

Check off the circles in the food group servings above as you record food and beverage items in the table at left. For sweets, give your best estimate of the total number of calories for the day.

**TODAY'S DATE:**

**TODAY'S GOAL:**

**NOTES ABOUT TODAY:**

**WHAT I ATE TODAY:**

Number of servings per food group

| Time | Food item | Amount | V | F | C | PD | Ft | S |
|------|-----------|--------|---|---|---|----|----|---|
|  |  |  |  |  |  |  |  |  |
|  |  |  |  |  |  |  |  |  |
|  |  |  |  |  |  |  |  |  |
|  |  |  |  |  |  |  |  |  |
|  |  |  |  |  |  |  |  |  |
|  |  |  |  |  |  |  |  |  |
|  |  |  |  |  |  |  |  |  |
|  |  |  |  |  |  |  |  |  |
|  |  |  |  |  |  |  |  |  |
|  |  |  |  |  |  |  |  |  |
|  |  |  |  |  |  |  |  |  |
|  |  |  |  |  |  |  |  |  |

**TODAY'S ACTIVITIES:**

🕐 Time

| | |
|---|---|
| | |
| | |
| | |
| | |
| **Total time (in minutes)** | |

**MOTIVATION TIP:**
Keeping a positive attitude about exercise is important for success. If you start thinking, "Exercise is boring" or "Exercise takes too much time," you'll quickly lose motivation.

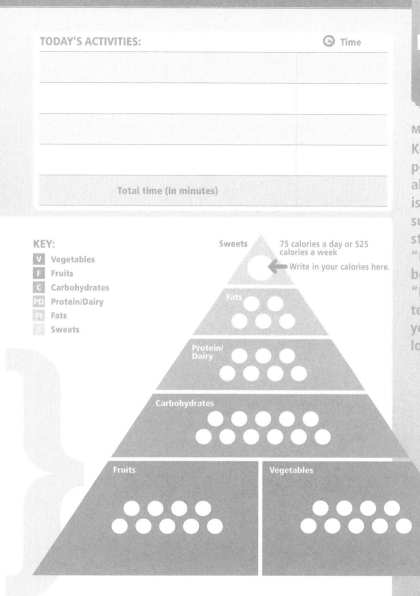

**KEY:**
- V Vegetables
- F Fruits
- C Carbohydrates
- PD Protein/Dairy
- R Fats
- S Sweets

Sweets
75 calories a day or 525 calories a week
Write in your calories here.

Fats

Protein/Dairy

Carbohydrates

Fruits

Vegetables

**WHAT I ATE TODAY FROM THE PYRAMID:**
Check off the circles in the food group servings above as you record food and beverage items in the table at left. For sweets, give your best estimate of the total number of calories for the day.

**TODAY'S DATE:**

**TODAY'S GOAL:**

**NOTES ABOUT TODAY:**
It's weigh-in day ~ record my weight in the weekly Review and the Weight Record.

**WHAT I ATE TODAY:**

Number of servings per food group

| Time | Food item | Amount | V | F | C | PD | Ft | S |
|------|-----------|--------|---|---|---|----|----|----|
|  |  |  |  |  |  |  |  |  |
|  |  |  |  |  |  |  |  |  |
|  |  |  |  |  |  |  |  |  |
|  |  |  |  |  |  |  |  |  |
|  |  |  |  |  |  |  |  |  |
|  |  |  |  |  |  |  |  |  |
|  |  |  |  |  |  |  |  |  |
|  |  |  |  |  |  |  |  |  |
|  |  |  |  |  |  |  |  |  |
|  |  |  |  |  |  |  |  |  |
|  |  |  |  |  |  |  |  |  |
|  |  |  |  |  |  |  |  |  |
|  |  |  |  |  |  |  |  |  |

## TODAY'S ACTIVITIES:

🕐 Time

| | |
|---|---|
| | |
| | |
| | |
| **Total time (in minutes)** | |

**REMINDER:**
Record your weight for today in the weekly Review and the Weight Record.

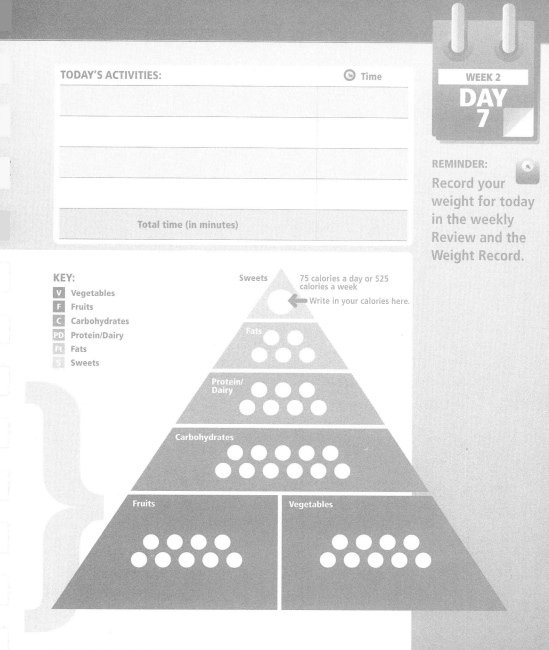

**KEY:**
- **V** Vegetables
- **F** Fruits
- **C** Carbohydrates
- **PD** Protein/Dairy
- **R** Fats
- **S** Sweets

Sweets — 75 calories a day or 525 calories a week
Write in your calories here.

Fats

Protein/Dairy

Carbohydrates

Fruits

Vegetables

## WHAT I ATE TODAY FROM THE PYRAMID:
Check off the circles in the food group servings above as you record food and beverage items in the table at left. For sweets, give your best estimate of the total number of calories for the day.

**My start weight** _____

**Minus my weight today** _____

**= Equals my weight change** _____

**I FEEL:**
- Terrific
- Good
- So-so
- Discouraged
- Like giving up

**I'M MOST PROUD OF:**

## WHAT WORKED WELL:

## WHAT DIDN'T WORK AS WELL:

## DID I REACH MY SERVINGS GOALS FOR THIS WEEK?

| Food group | Daily servings | Day 1 | Day 2 | Day 3 | Day 4 | Day 5 | Day 6 | Day 7 |
|---|---|---|---|---|---|---|---|---|
| Vegetables | | ○ | ○ | ○ | ○ | ○ | ○ | ○ |
| Fruits | | ○ | ○ | ○ | ○ | ○ | ○ | ○ |
| Carbohydrates | | ○ | ○ | ○ | ○ | ○ | ○ | ○ |
| Protein/Dairy | | ○ | ○ | ○ | ○ | ○ | ○ | ○ |
| Fats | | ○ | ○ | ○ | ○ | ○ | ○ | ○ |
| Sweets | | ○ | ○ | ○ | ○ | ○ | ○ | ○ |

## DIRECTIONS:

1. Write your daily serving goals for each food group in the table above.
2. Compare the serving totals that you recorded for each day of the past week with your goals.
3. Check off the circles in the table above if your serving totals have met your goals.

**NEW FOOD I WOULD LIKE TO TRY:**

**NEW WAYS TO ADD ACTIVITY TO MY DAY:**

**REMINDER:**
Calculate your weight change in this Review and record it in the Weight Record.

## HOW MANY STEPS A DAY DID I TAKE (IF I USED A PEDOMETER)?

| Day 1 | Day 2 | Day 3 | Day 4 | Day 5 | Day 6 | Day 7 |
|-------|-------|-------|-------|-------|-------|-------|
|       |       |       |       |       |       |       |

## HOW MANY MINUTES A DAY WAS I ACTIVE?

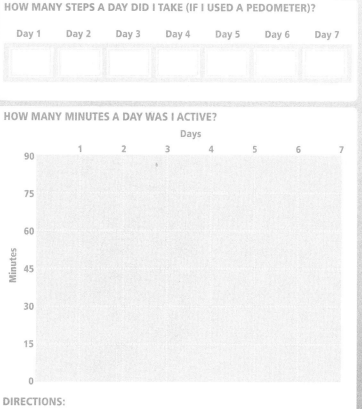

**DIRECTIONS:**
1. Add a dot for your total minutes of activity for each day of last week.
2. Connect each dot on the chart with a line.

See a sample chart to the right. →

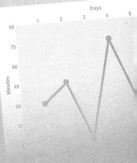

DID I REACH MY SERVINGS GOALS FOR THI...

| Food group | Daily servings | Day 1 |
|------------|----------------|-------|
| Vegetables | 4+ | ✓ |
| Fruits | 3+ | |
| Carbohydrates | 4 | ✓ |
| Protein/Dairy | 3 | ✓ |
| Fats | 5 | |

The samples above show how you can fill out your servings goals table and your activity chart for your weekly Review.

| Day | Breakfast | Lunch | Dinner | Snack |
|---|---|---|---|---|
| EXAMPLE | cereal banana | spaghetti fruit salad | tuna wrap baby carrots | crackers and cheese |
| 1 | | | | |
| 2 | | | | |
| 3 | | | | |
| 4 | | | | |
| 5 | | | | |
| 6 | | | | |
| 7 | | | | |

| Exercise and activities | Events and special plans |
|---|---|
| swim class @ 11am<br>walk to work | kids ballgame @ 6pm<br>note: supper will be on the go |
| | |
| | |
| | |
| | |
| | |
| | |
| | |

# WEEK AT A GLANCE

**USING THE PLANNER:**

Organize your plans for meals, activities and exercise in the coming week. Note upcoming events that may affect your weight program, such as travel, eating out, social occasions and vacations.

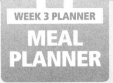

| MAIN MEAL OR MEALS OF THE DAY | HOW MUCH |
|---|---|
| | |

**EASY AS 1, 2, 3:**

This page allows you to check how well a meal meets your recommended servings goals.

1. Write down what you're planning to eat for this meal (or for the entire day).
2. Calculate the number of servings based on how much you're planning to eat.
3. Be sure to include the food items from your menu in your Shopping List.

## PYRAMID SERVINGS FOR THIS MEAL

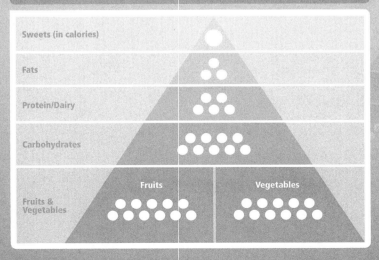

◄ Check off the number of servings on the pyramid at left.

| MAIN MEAL OR MEALS OF THE DAY | HOW MUCH |
|---|---|
|  |  |

**EASY AS 1, 2, 3:**

This page allows you to check how well a meal meets your recommended servings goals.

1. Write down what you're planning to eat for this meal (or for the entire day).
2. Calculate the number of servings based on how much you're planning to eat.
3. Be sure to include the food items from your menu in your Shopping List.

## PYRAMID SERVINGS FOR THIS MEAL

Sweets (in calories)

Fats

Protein/Dairy

Carbohydrates

Fruits & Vegetables

Fruits

Vegetables

75

◄ Check off the number of servings on the pyramid at left.

## MENU FOR THE DAY

### BREAKFAST
1 whole-grain bagel
3 tbsp. fat-free cream cheese
*1 medium orange
Calorie-free beverage

| V | F | C | PD | Ft | S |
|---|---|---|----|----|---|
| 0 | 1 | 2 | 0  | 1  | 0 |

### LUNCH
Smoked Turkey Wrap
Cucumber and Tomato Salad
*1 small apple
Calorie-free beverage

| V | F | C | PD | Ft | S |
|---|---|---|----|----|---|
| 2 | 1 | 1 | 1  | 1  | 0 |

### DINNER
1 serving Beef Kebab
3 baby, red-skinned potatoes
*1 large kiwi fruit
Calorie-free beverage

| V | F | C | PD | Ft | S |
|---|---|---|----|----|---|
| 2 | 1 | 1 | 2  | 0  | 0 |

### SNACK
*1 serving favorite vegetable
2 tbsp. reduced-calorie vegetable dip

| V | F | C | PD | Ft | S |
|---|---|---|----|----|---|
| 1 | 0 | 0 | 0  | 1  | 0 |

*The serving size stated is the minimum amount. Eat as much as you wish.

QUICK TIP:

The menu on this page demonstrates how you can plan your own daily menus. Feel free to include this sample on one of your days.

### LUNCH RECIPE

## Smoked Turkey Wrap

- Place 3 ounces of thin-sliced smoked turkey, shredded lettuce, sliced tomato and onion on a 6-inch tortilla. Top with 2 tablespoons of reduced-calorie Western dressing. Roll up tortilla.

### LUNCH RECIPE

## Cucumber and Tomato Salad

- Combine 1 cup of thinly sliced cucumber and 8 cherry tomatoes, halved. Add balsamic, rice wine or herb-flavored vinegar to taste.

### DINNER RECIPE

## Beef Kebabs

- Place 3 ounces of marinated cubed round steak and a total of 2 cups diced fresh mushrooms, tomatoes, green peppers and onions on skewers. Broil or grill.

| Fresh produce | Whole grains | Meat & dairy |
| --- | --- | --- |
| | | |

| Frozen goods | Canned goods | Miscellaneous |
| --- | --- | --- |
| | | |

**QUICK TIP:**

Create your shopping list for the week before going to the grocery store. You'll have all the ingredients on hand at the time you prepare a meal.

| Fresh produce | Whole grain |
| --- | --- |
| 10 large tomatoes | 8 oz package spaghetti |
| 2 red peppers | 1 loaf rye brea |
| summer squash | 1 package en muffins |
| zucchini | |
| 1 bag baby carrots | bag of pita |
| cherries | |
| 3 grapefruit | |

Add to your Shopping List as you plan your menus for the week.

**TODAY'S DATE:**

**TODAY'S GOAL:**

**NOTES ABOUT TODAY:**

**WHAT I ATE TODAY:**

Number of servings per food group

| 🕐 Time | Food item | Amount | V | F | C | PD | Ft | S |
|---------|-----------|--------|---|---|---|----|----|----|
|         |           |        |   |   |   |    |    |    |
|         |           |        |   |   |   |    |    |    |
|         |           |        |   |   |   |    |    |    |
|         |           |        |   |   |   |    |    |    |
|         |           |        |   |   |   |    |    |    |
|         |           |        |   |   |   |    |    |    |
|         |           |        |   |   |   |    |    |    |
|         |           |        |   |   |   |    |    |    |
|         |           |        |   |   |   |    |    |    |
|         |           |        |   |   |   |    |    |    |
|         |           |        |   |   |   |    |    |    |

**TODAY'S ACTIVITIES:**                                     🕐 Time

|  |  |
|---|---|
|  |  |
|  |  |
|  |  |
|  |  |
| **Total time (in minutes)** |  |

**MOTIVATION TIP:**
Don't get hung up on exact servings totals for a day. Think in terms of the week as well. For example, if on one day you don't reach your target for fruit servings, you can always add extra servings on the next day.

**KEY:**
- **V** Vegetables
- **F** Fruits
- **C** Carbohydrates
- **PD** Protein/Dairy
- **Ft** Fats
- **S** Sweets

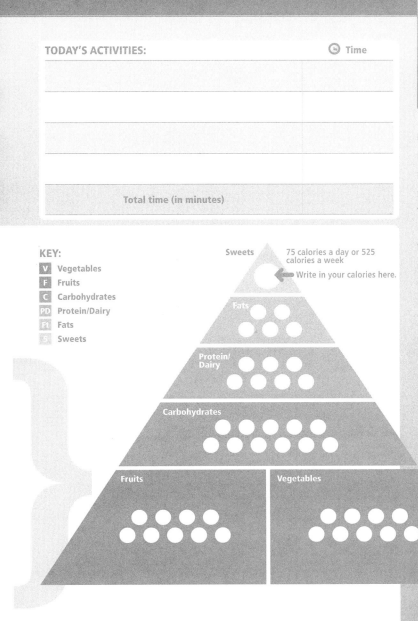

Sweets — 75 calories a day or 525 calories a week
→ Write in your calories here.

**WHAT I ATE TODAY FROM THE PYRAMID:**
Check off the circles in the food group servings above as you record food and beverage items in the table at left. For sweets, give your best estimate of the total number of calories for the day.

**TODAY'S DATE:**

**TODAY'S GOAL:**

**NOTES ABOUT TODAY:**

**WHAT I ATE TODAY:**                           Number of servings per food group

| Time | Food item | Amount | V | F | C | PD | Ft | S |
|------|-----------|--------|---|---|---|----|----|----|
|  |  |  |  |  |  |  |  |  |
|  |  |  |  |  |  |  |  |  |
|  |  |  |  |  |  |  |  |  |
|  |  |  |  |  |  |  |  |  |
|  |  |  |  |  |  |  |  |  |
|  |  |  |  |  |  |  |  |  |
|  |  |  |  |  |  |  |  |  |
|  |  |  |  |  |  |  |  |  |
|  |  |  |  |  |  |  |  |  |
|  |  |  |  |  |  |  |  |  |
|  |  |  |  |  |  |  |  |  |
|  |  |  |  |  |  |  |  |  |

**TODAY'S ACTIVITIES:**

🕐 Time

|  |  |
|---|---|
|  |  |
|  |  |
|  |  |
| **Total time (in minutes)** |  |

**MOTIVATION TIP:**
Rather than dwell on what you can't eat, focus on what you can eat. Granted, you may no longer be able to eat a large bowl of ice cream every evening, but you can have ice cream on occasion.

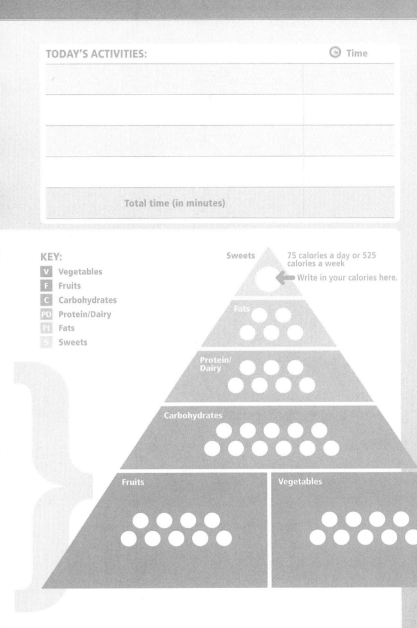

**KEY:**
- V  Vegetables
- F  Fruits
- C  Carbohydrates
- PD  Protein/Dairy
- Ft  Fats
- S  Sweets

Sweets
75 calories a day or 525 calories a week
Write in your calories here.

Fats

Protein/Dairy

Carbohydrates

Fruits

Vegetables

**WHAT I ATE TODAY FROM THE PYRAMID:**
Check off the circles in the food group servings above as you record food and beverage items in the table at left. For sweets, give your best estimate of the total number of calories for the day.

**TODAY'S DATE:**

**TODAY'S GOAL:**

**NOTES ABOUT TODAY:**

**WHAT I ATE TODAY:**                                                    Number of servings per food group

| 🕐 Time | Food item | Amount | V | F | C | PD | Ft | S |
|---------|-----------|--------|---|---|---|----|----|---|
|         |           |        |   |   |   |    |    |   |
|         |           |        |   |   |   |    |    |   |
|         |           |        |   |   |   |    |    |   |
|         |           |        |   |   |   |    |    |   |
|         |           |        |   |   |   |    |    |   |
|         |           |        |   |   |   |    |    |   |
|         |           |        |   |   |   |    |    |   |
|         |           |        |   |   |   |    |    |   |
|         |           |        |   |   |   |    |    |   |
|         |           |        |   |   |   |    |    |   |

**TODAY'S ACTIVITIES:**                                              🕐 Time

Total time (in minutes)

**MOTIVATION TIP:**

If your schedule is full, you can still find time to exercise for brief periods during the day. For example, do three 10-minute sessions in place of one 30-minute session.

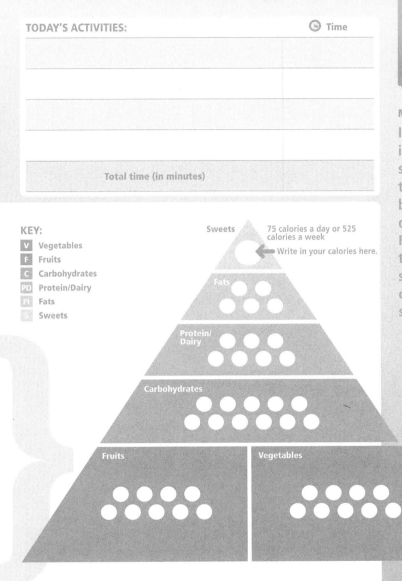

**KEY:**
- V Vegetables
- F Fruits
- C Carbohydrates
- PD Protein/Dairy
- R Fats
- S Sweets

Sweets    75 calories a day or 525 calories a week
← Write in your calories here.

Fats

Protein/ Dairy

Carbohydrates

Fruits

Vegetables

**WHAT I ATE TODAY FROM THE PYRAMID:**

Check off the circles in the food group servings above as you record food and beverage items in the table at left. For sweets, give your best estimate of the total number of calories for the day.

**TODAY'S DATE:**

**TODAY'S GOAL:**

**NOTES ABOUT TODAY:**

**WHAT I ATE TODAY:**

Number of servings per food group

| ⏱ Time | Food item | Amount | V | F | C | PD | Ft | S |
|--------|-----------|--------|---|---|---|----|----|----|
|  |  |  |  |  |  |  |  |  |
|  |  |  |  |  |  |  |  |  |
|  |  |  |  |  |  |  |  |  |
|  |  |  |  |  |  |  |  |  |
|  |  |  |  |  |  |  |  |  |
|  |  |  |  |  |  |  |  |  |
|  |  |  |  |  |  |  |  |  |
|  |  |  |  |  |  |  |  |  |
|  |  |  |  |  |  |  |  |  |
|  |  |  |  |  |  |  |  |  |
|  |  |  |  |  |  |  |  |  |
|  |  |  |  |  |  |  |  |  |

**TODAY'S ACTIVITIES:**

🕐 Time

Total time (in minutes)

**MOTIVATION TIP:**
Give yourself some slack. For example, it's OK to take a day off from exercising now and then — if you feel you really need it. You're not in exercise boot camp.

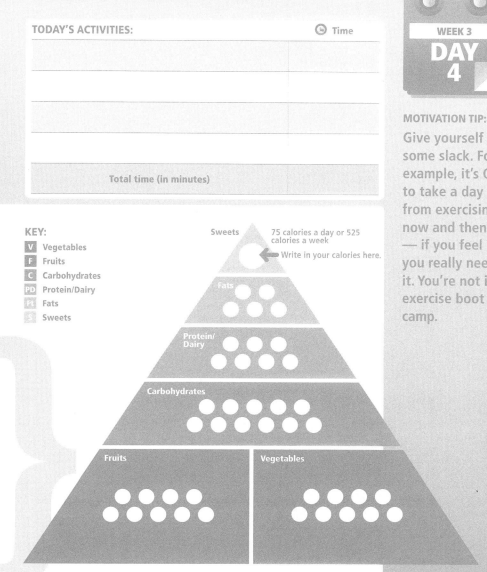

**KEY:**
- V Vegetables
- F Fruits
- C Carbohydrates
- PD Protein/Dairy
- F Fats
- S Sweets

Sweets — 75 calories a day or 525 calories a week
← Write in your calories here.

Fats

Protein/Dairy

Carbohydrates

Fruits

Vegetables

**WHAT I ATE TODAY FROM THE PYRAMID:**
Check off the circles in the food group servings above as you record food and beverage items in the table at left. For sweets, give your best estimate of the total number of calories for the day.

**TODAY'S DATE:**

**TODAY'S GOAL:**

**NOTES ABOUT TODAY:**

**WHAT I ATE TODAY:**

**Number of servings per food group**

| Time | Food item | Amount | V | F | C | PD | Ft | S |
|------|-----------|--------|---|---|---|----|----|---|
|      |           |        |   |   |   |    |    |   |
|      |           |        |   |   |   |    |    |   |
|      |           |        |   |   |   |    |    |   |
|      |           |        |   |   |   |    |    |   |
|      |           |        |   |   |   |    |    |   |
|      |           |        |   |   |   |    |    |   |
|      |           |        |   |   |   |    |    |   |
|      |           |        |   |   |   |    |    |   |
|      |           |        |   |   |   |    |    |   |
|      |           |        |   |   |   |    |    |   |
|      |           |        |   |   |   |    |    |   |
|      |           |        |   |   |   |    |    |   |

**TODAY'S ACTIVITIES:** 🕐 **Time**

Total time (in minutes)

**MOTIVATION TIP:**
Be happy with who you are and not who you imagine yourself being. Think of a skill or talent that you take special pride in. Then fill in the blank, "I like the fact that I can _____."

**KEY:**
- **V** Vegetables
- **F** Fruits
- **C** Carbohydrates
- **PD** Protein/Dairy
- **FL** Fats
- **S** Sweets

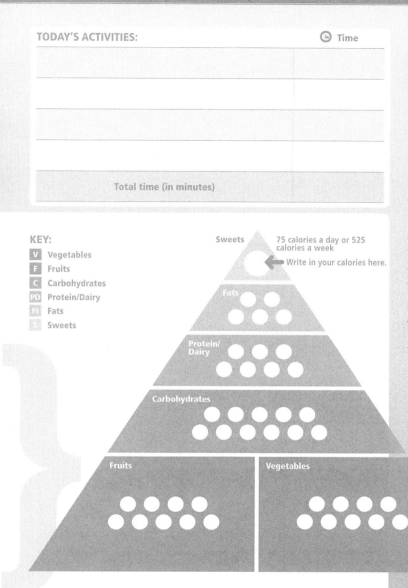

Sweets — 75 calories a day or 525 calories a week
← Write in your calories here.

Fats

Protein/Dairy

Carbohydrates

Fruits

Vegetables

**WHAT I ATE TODAY FROM THE PYRAMID:**
Check off the circles in the food group servings above as you record food and beverage items in the table at left. For sweets, give your best estimate of the total number of calories for the day.

**TODAY'S DATE:**

**TODAY'S GOAL:**

**NOTES ABOUT TODAY:**

**WHAT I ATE TODAY:**     Number of servings per food group

| Time | Food item | Amount | V | F | C | PD | Ft | S |
|------|-----------|--------|---|---|---|----|----|----|
| | | | | | | | | |
| | | | | | | | | |
| | | | | | | | | |
| | | | | | | | | |
| | | | | | | | | |
| | | | | | | | | |
| | | | | | | | | |
| | | | | | | | | |
| | | | | | | | | |
| | | | | | | | | |
| | | | | | | | | |
| | | | | | | | | |

**TODAY'S ACTIVITIES:**

🕐 **Time**

Total time (in minutes)

Test your menu skills. Carefully review items and look for terms that may indicate how the food is prepared or what ingredients may be included. Try to identify sources of hidden calories.

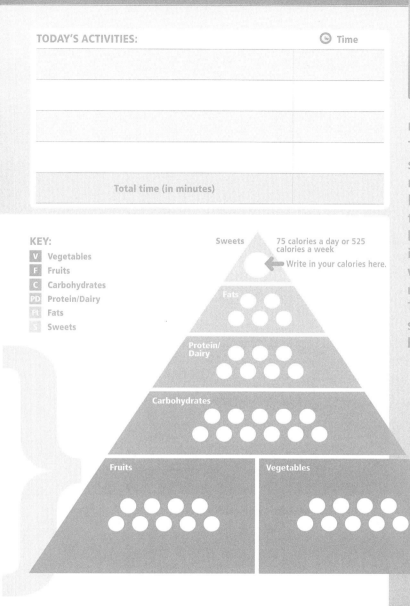

**KEY:**

- V Vegetables
- F Fruits
- C Carbohydrates
- PD Protein/Dairy
- Ft Fats
- S Sweets

Sweets — 75 calories a day or 525 calories a week

← Write in your calories here.

Fats

Protein/Dairy

Carbohydrates

Fruits

Vegetables

**WHAT I ATE TODAY FROM THE PYRAMID:**

Check off the circles in the food group servings above as you record food and beverage items in the table at left. For sweets, give your best estimate of the total number of calories for the day.

**TODAY'S DATE:**

**TODAY'S GOAL:**

**NOTES ABOUT TODAY:**
It's weigh-in day ~ record my weight in the weekly Review and the Weight Record.

**WHAT I ATE TODAY:**

| ⊙ Time | Food item | Amount | V | F | C | PD | Pt | S |
|--------|-----------|--------|---|---|---|----|----|---|
| | | | | | | | | |
| | | | | | | | | |
| | | | | | | | | |
| | | | | | | | | |
| | | | | | | | | |
| | | | | | | | | |
| | | | | | | | | |
| | | | | | | | | |
| | | | | | | | | |
| | | | | | | | | |
| | | | | | | | | |
| | | | | | | | | |
| | | | | | | | | |
| | | | | | | | | |

Number of servings per food group

**TODAY'S ACTIVITIES:**

🕐 Time

Total time (in minutes)

**REMINDER:**
Record your weight for today in the weekly Review and the Weight Record.

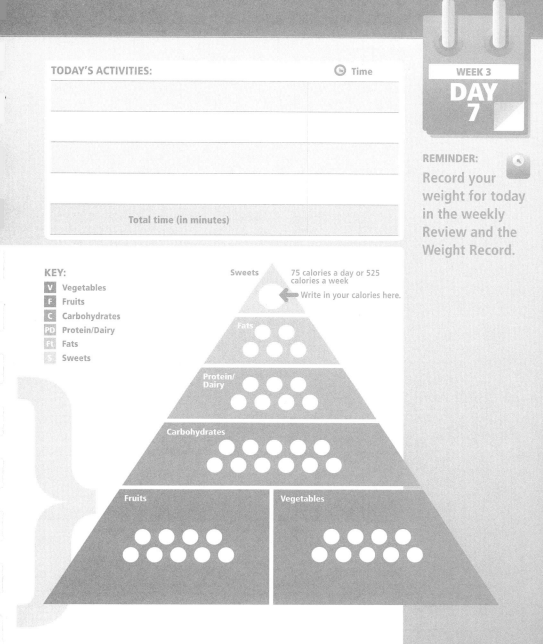

**KEY:**

**V** Vegetables
**F** Fruits
**C** Carbohydrates
**PD** Protein/Dairy
**Ft** Fats
**S** Sweets

Sweets — 75 calories a day or 525 calories a week

← Write in your calories here.

Fats

Protein/Dairy

Carbohydrates

Fruits

Vegetables

**WHAT I ATE TODAY FROM THE PYRAMID:**
Check off the circles in the food group servings above as you record food and beverage items in the table at left. For sweets, give your best estimate of the total number of calories for the day.

| My start weight | | I FEEL: | I'M MOST PROUD OF: |
|---|---|---|---|
| Minus my weight today | | ○ Terrific | |
| = Equals my weight change | | ○ Good | |
| | | ○ So-so | |
| | | ○ Discouraged | |
| | | ○ Like giving up | |

**WHAT WORKED WELL:**

**WHAT DIDN'T WORK AS WELL:**

**DID I REACH MY SERVINGS GOALS FOR THIS WEEK?**

| Food group | Daily servings | Day 1 | Day 2 | Day 3 | Day 4 | Day 5 | Day 6 | Day 7 |
|---|---|---|---|---|---|---|---|---|
| Vegetables | | ○ | ○ | ○ | ○ | ○ | ○ | ○ |
| Fruits | | ○ | ○ | ○ | ○ | ○ | ○ | ○ |
| Carbohydrates | | ○ | ○ | ○ | ○ | ○ | ○ | ○ |
| Protein/Dairy | | ○ | ○ | ○ | ○ | ○ | ○ | ○ |
| Fats | | ○ | ○ | ○ | ○ | ○ | ○ | ○ |
| Sweets | | ○ | ○ | ○ | ○ | ○ | ○ | ○ |

**DIRECTIONS:**

1. Write your daily serving goals for each food group in the table above.
2. Compare the serving totals that you recorded for each day of the past week with your goals.
3. Check off the circles in the table above if your serving totals have met your goals.

**NEW FOOD I WOULD LIKE TO TRY:**

**NEW WAYS TO ADD ACTIVITY TO MY DAY:**

**HOW MANY STEPS A DAY DID I TAKE (IF I USED A PEDOMETER)?**

| Day 1 | Day 2 | Day 3 | Day 4 | Day 5 | Day 6 | Day 7 |
|-------|-------|-------|-------|-------|-------|-------|
|       |       |       |       |       |       |       |

**REMINDER:**
Calculate your weight change in this Review and record it in the Weight Record.

**HOW MANY MINUTES A DAY WAS I ACTIVE?**

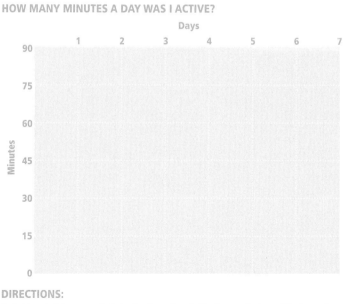

**DIRECTIONS:**

1. Add a dot for your total minutes of activity for each day of last week.
2. Connect each dot on the chart with a line.

See a sample chart to the right. →

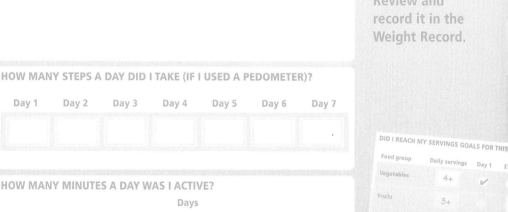

| DID I REACH MY SERVINGS GOALS FOR THIS | | |
|---|---|---|
| Food group | Daily servings | Day 1 |
| Vegetables | 4+ | ✓ |
| Fruits | 3+ | |
| Carbohydrates | 4 | ✓ |
| Protein/Dairy | 3 | ✓ |
| Fats | 5 | |

The samples above show how you can fill out your servings goals table and your activity chart for your weekly Review.

| Day | Breakfast | Lunch | Dinner | Snack |
|---|---|---|---|---|
| EXAMPLE | cereal<br>banana | spaghetti<br>fruit salad | tuna wrap<br>baby carrots | crackers<br>and cheese |
| 1 | | | | |
| 2 | | | | |
| 3 | | | | |
| 4 | | | | |
| 5 | | | | |
| 6 | | | | |
| 7 | | | | |

| Exercise and activities | Events and special plans |
|---|---|
| swim class @ 11am<br>walk to work | kids ballgame @ 6pm<br>note: supper will be on the go |
| | |
| | |
| | |
| | |
| | |
| | |
| | |

**USING THE PLANNER:**

Organize your plans for meals, activities and exercise in the coming week. Note upcoming events that may affect your weight program, such as travel, eating out, social occasions and vacations.

| MAIN MEAL OR MEALS OF THE DAY | HOW MUCH |
|---|---|
| | |

**EASY AS 1, 2, 3:**

This page allows you to check how well a meal meets your recommended servings goals.

1. Write down what you're planning to eat for this meal (or for the entire day).
2. Calculate the number of servings based on how much you're planning to eat.
3. Be sure to include the food items from your menu in your Shopping List.

## PYRAMID SERVINGS FOR THIS MEAL

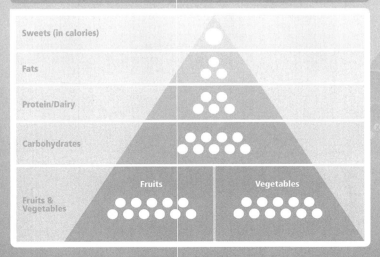

◄ Check off the number of servings on the pyramid at left.

WEEK 4 PLANNER

# MEAL PLANNER

| MAIN MEAL OR MEALS OF THE DAY | HOW MUCH |
|---|---|
| | |

## EASY AS 1, 2, 3:

This page allows you to check how well a meal meets your recommended servings goals.

1. Write down what you're planning to eat for this meal (or for the entire day).

2. Calculate the number of servings based on how much you're planning to eat.

3. Be sure to include the food items from your menu in your Shopping List.

## PYRAMID SERVINGS FOR THIS MEAL

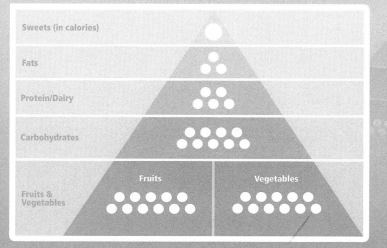

Sweets (in calories)

Fats

Protein/Dairy

Carbohydrates

Fruits & Vegetables

Fruits

Vegetables

75

◄ Check off the number of servings on the pyramid at left.

## MENU FOR THE DAY

### BREAKFAST
½ c. cooked oatmeal
2 tbsp. raisins
1 c. skim milk
Calorie-free beverage

| V | F | C | PD | Ft | S |
|---|---|---|----|----|---|
| 0 | 2 | 1 | 1 | 0 | 0 |

### LUNCH
Southwestern Salad
½ whole-grain pita bread
Calorie-free beverage

| V | F | C | PD | Ft | S |
|---|---|---|----|----|---|
| 2 | 1 | 1 | 1 | 2 | 0 |

### DINNER
¼ Classic Tomato-Basil Pizza
*½ c. baby carrots
*¼ small cantaloupe
Calorie-free beverage

| V | F | C | PD | Ft | S |
|---|---|---|----|----|---|
| 2 | 1 | 2 | 1 | 0 | 0 |

### SNACK
7 whole almonds

| V | F | C | PD | Ft | S |
|---|---|---|----|----|---|
| 0 | 0 | 0 | 0 | 1 | 0 |

*The serving size stated is the minimum amount. Eat as much as you wish.

QUICK TIP:

**The menu on this page demonstrates how you can plan your own daily menus. Feel free to include this sample on one of your days.**

### LUNCH RECIPE

## Southwestern Salad

- Top 2 cups shredded lettuce with 2½ ounces shredded cooked chicken, 1 cup chopped green peppers and onions, ½ cup crushed pineapple, ⅙ avocado and 2 tablespoons of reduced-calorie Western dressing.

### DINNER RECIPE

## Classic Tomato-Basil Pizza

- Top a prepared 12-inch pizza crust with 1 cup diced plum tomatoes, fresh basil and 1⅓ cup low-fat shredded mozzarella cheese. Bake at 400 F about 10 minutes.

**WEEK 4 PLANNER**
# SHOPPING LIST

| Fresh produce | Whole grains | Meat & dairy |
|---|---|---|
| | | |

| Frozen goods | Canned goods | Miscellaneous |
|---|---|---|
| | | |

QUICK TIP:

Create your shopping list for the week before going to the grocery store. You'll have all the ingredients on hand at the time you prepare a meal.

| Fresh produce | Whole grains |
|---|---|
| 10 large tomatoes | 8 oz package spaghetti |
| 2 red peppers | 1 loaf rye bread |
| summer squash | 1 package eng muffins |
| zucchini | |
| 1 bag baby carrots | bag of pita |
| cherries | |
| 3 grapefruit | |

Add to your Shopping List as you plan your menus for the week.

**TODAY'S DATE:**

**TODAY'S GOAL:**

**NOTES ABOUT TODAY:**

**WHAT I ATE TODAY:**

Number of servings per food group

| 🕐 Time | Food item | Amount | V | F | C | PD | Ft | S |
|---------|-----------|--------|---|---|---|----|----|---|
|         |           |        |   |   |   |    |    |   |
|         |           |        |   |   |   |    |    |   |
|         |           |        |   |   |   |    |    |   |
|         |           |        |   |   |   |    |    |   |
|         |           |        |   |   |   |    |    |   |
|         |           |        |   |   |   |    |    |   |
|         |           |        |   |   |   |    |    |   |
|         |           |        |   |   |   |    |    |   |
|         |           |        |   |   |   |    |    |   |
|         |           |        |   |   |   |    |    |   |
|         |           |        |   |   |   |    |    |   |

**TODAY'S ACTIVITIES:**

**Time**

Total time (in minutes)

**MOTIVATION TIP:**
Try not to focus only on physical exertion while you exercise. Think of pleasant thoughts or enjoyable things to do at the same time that you're physically active.

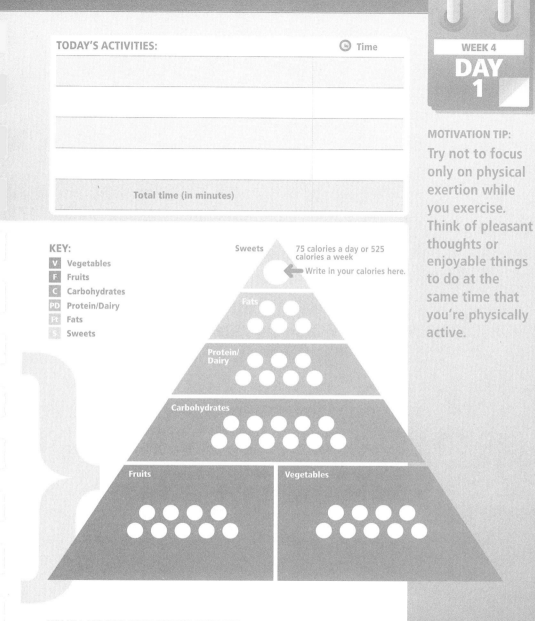

**KEY:**
- **V** Vegetables
- **F** Fruits
- **C** Carbohydrates
- **PD** Protein/Dairy
- **Ft** Fats
- **S** Sweets

**Sweets**
75 calories a day or 525 calories a week
Write in your calories here.

**Fats**

**Protein/Dairy**

**Carbohydrates**

**Fruits**

**Vegetables**

**WHAT I ATE TODAY FROM THE PYRAMID:**
Check off the circles in the food group servings above as you record food and beverage items in the table at left. For sweets, give your best estimate of the total number of calories for the day.

**TODAY'S DATE:**

**TODAY'S GOAL:**

**NOTES ABOUT TODAY:**

## WHAT I ATE TODAY:

Number of servings per food group

| Time | Food item | Amount | V | F | C | PD | Ft | S |
|------|-----------|--------|---|---|---|----|----|---|
|      |           |        |   |   |   |    |    |   |
|      |           |        |   |   |   |    |    |   |
|      |           |        |   |   |   |    |    |   |
|      |           |        |   |   |   |    |    |   |
|      |           |        |   |   |   |    |    |   |
|      |           |        |   |   |   |    |    |   |
|      |           |        |   |   |   |    |    |   |
|      |           |        |   |   |   |    |    |   |
|      |           |        |   |   |   |    |    |   |
|      |           |        |   |   |   |    |    |   |
|      |           |        |   |   |   |    |    |   |

## TODAY'S ACTIVITIES:

⏱ Time

Total time (in minutes)

MOTIVATION TIP:
The urge to eat can often be due to a certain mood and not to physical hunger. When the mood sets in, try to distract yourself by going for a walk, calling a friend or running an errand.

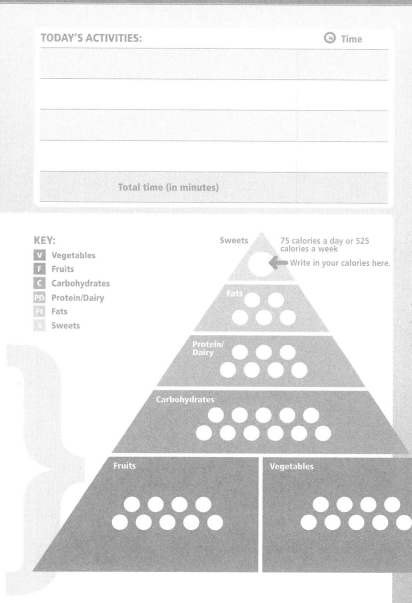

KEY:
- V  Vegetables
- F  Fruits
- C  Carbohydrates
- PD  Protein/Dairy
- Ft  Fats
- S  Sweets

Sweets — 75 calories a day or 525 calories a week
Write in your calories here.

Fats

Protein/Dairy

Carbohydrates

Fruits

Vegetables

## WHAT I ATE TODAY FROM THE PYRAMID:
Check off the circles in the food group servings above as you record food and beverage items in the table at left. For sweets, give your best estimate of the total number of calories for the day.

**TODAY'S DATE:**

**TODAY'S GOAL:**

**NOTES ABOUT TODAY:**

**WHAT I ATE TODAY:**       Number of servings per food group

| ⏱ Time | Food item | Amount | V | F | C | PD | Ft | ⟩ |
|---|---|---|---|---|---|---|---|---|
|  |  |  |  |  |  |  |  |  |
|  |  |  |  |  |  |  |  |  |
|  |  |  |  |  |  |  |  |  |
|  |  |  |  |  |  |  |  |  |
|  |  |  |  |  |  |  |  |  |
|  |  |  |  |  |  |  |  |  |
|  |  |  |  |  |  |  |  |  |
|  |  |  |  |  |  |  |  |  |
|  |  |  |  |  |  |  |  |  |
|  |  |  |  |  |  |  |  |  |
|  |  |  |  |  |  |  |  |  |
|  |  |  |  |  |  |  |  |  |

**TODAY'S ACTIVITIES:**                              🕐 Time

Total time (in minutes)

**MOTIVATION TIP:**
Accept the fact that on some days, you'll have setbacks. Rather than give up on your program entirely, simply start fresh on the next day. Believe in yourself.

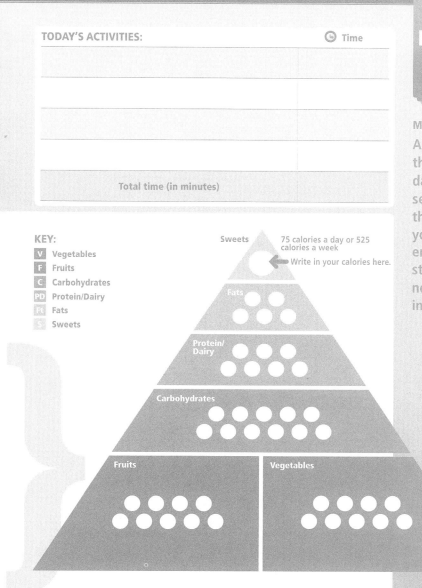

**KEY:**
- V Vegetables
- F Fruits
- C Carbohydrates
- PD Protein/Dairy
- Ft Fats
- S Sweets

Sweets — 75 calories a day or 525 calories a week
Write in your calories here.

Fats

Protein/Dairy

Carbohydrates

Fruits

Vegetables

**WHAT I ATE TODAY FROM THE PYRAMID:**
Check off the circles in the food group servings above as you record food and beverage items in the table at left. For sweets, give your best estimate of the total number of calories for the day.

**TODAY'S DATE:**

**TODAY'S GOAL:**

**NOTES ABOUT TODAY:**

**WHAT I ATE TODAY:**　　　　　　　　　　　Number of servings per food group

| Time | Food item | Amount | V | F | C | PD | Ft | S |
|------|-----------|--------|---|---|---|----|----|---|
| | | | | | | | | |
| | | | | | | | | |
| | | | | | | | | |
| | | | | | | | | |
| | | | | | | | | |
| | | | | | | | | |
| | | | | | | | | |
| | | | | | | | | |
| | | | | | | | | |
| | | | | | | | | |
| | | | | | | | | |
| | | | | | | | | |
| | | | | | | | | |

**TODAY'S ACTIVITIES:**

🕐 Time

Total time (in minutes)

**MOTIVATION TIP:**

You don't have to like all vegetables and fruits, just some of them. To increase the number of servings you eat, try preparing them in different ways, for example, grilling or making fruit smoothies.

**KEY:**

- V Vegetables
- F Fruits
- C Carbohydrates
- PD Protein/Dairy
- Ft Fats
- S Sweets

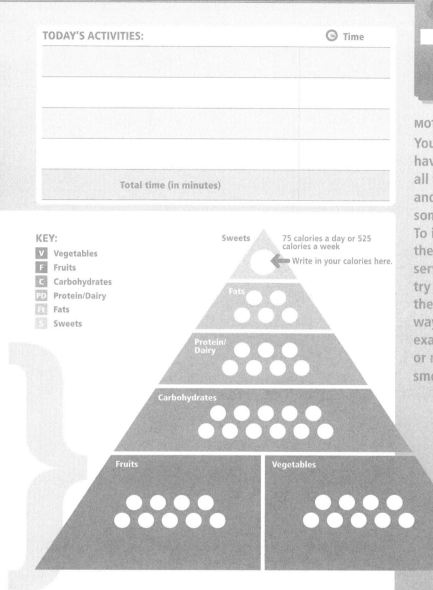

Sweets — 75 calories a day or 525 calories a week

Write in your calories here.

Fats

Protein/Dairy

Carbohydrates

Fruits

Vegetables

**WHAT I ATE TODAY FROM THE PYRAMID:**

Check off the circles in the food group servings above as you record food and beverage items in the table at left. For sweets, give your best estimate of the total number of calories for the day.

**TODAY'S DATE:**

**TODAY'S GOAL:**

**NOTES ABOUT TODAY:**

**WHAT I ATE TODAY:**

Number of servings per food group

| ⏱ Time | Food item | Amount | V | F | C | PD | Pt | S |
|---------|-----------|--------|---|---|---|----|----|---|
|         |           |        |   |   |   |    |    |   |
|         |           |        |   |   |   |    |    |   |
|         |           |        |   |   |   |    |    |   |
|         |           |        |   |   |   |    |    |   |
|         |           |        |   |   |   |    |    |   |
|         |           |        |   |   |   |    |    |   |
|         |           |        |   |   |   |    |    |   |
|         |           |        |   |   |   |    |    |   |
|         |           |        |   |   |   |    |    |   |
|         |           |        |   |   |   |    |    |   |
|         |           |        |   |   |   |    |    |   |
|         |           |        |   |   |   |    |    |   |
|         |           |        |   |   |   |    |    |   |

**TODAY'S ACTIVITIES:**     🕐 **Time**

Total time (in minutes)

**MOTIVATION TIP:**

Don't let unsupportive friends distract you from your goals. Try to be around people who share similar goals and who are willing to provide support.

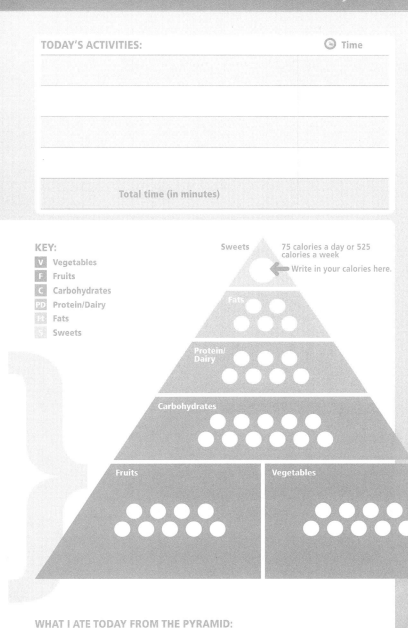

**KEY:**

- **V** Vegetables
- **F** Fruits
- **C** Carbohydrates
- **PD** Protein/Dairy
- **Ft** Fats
- **S** Sweets

Sweets    75 calories a day or 525 calories a week

Write in your calories here.

Fats

Protein/Dairy

Carbohydrates

Fruits        Vegetables

**WHAT I ATE TODAY FROM THE PYRAMID:**

Check off the circles in the food group servings above as you record food and beverage items in the table at left. For sweets, give your best estimate of the total number of calories for the day.

**TODAY'S DATE:**

**TODAY'S GOAL:**

**NOTES ABOUT TODAY:**

**WHAT I ATE TODAY:**                                                    Number of servings per food group

| Time | Food item | Amount | V | F | C | PD | Pt | S |
|------|-----------|--------|---|---|---|----|----|---|
|      |           |        |   |   |   |    |    |   |
|      |           |        |   |   |   |    |    |   |
|      |           |        |   |   |   |    |    |   |
|      |           |        |   |   |   |    |    |   |
|      |           |        |   |   |   |    |    |   |
|      |           |        |   |   |   |    |    |   |
|      |           |        |   |   |   |    |    |   |
|      |           |        |   |   |   |    |    |   |
|      |           |        |   |   |   |    |    |   |
|      |           |        |   |   |   |    |    |   |

TODAY'S ACTIVITIES:

🕐 Time

| | |
|---|---|
| | |
| | |
| | |
| | |
| **Total time (in minutes)** | |

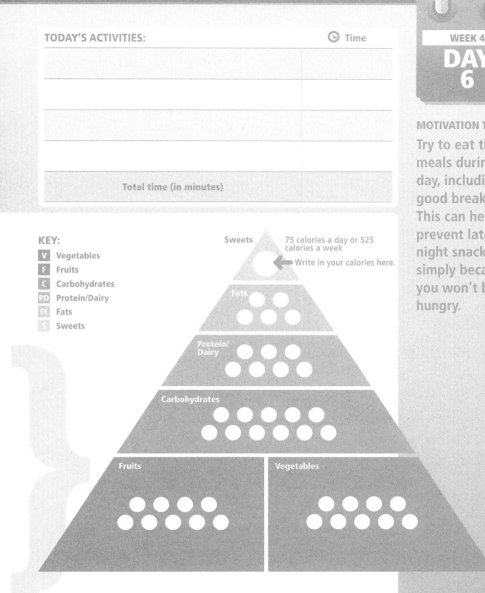

**KEY:**
- **V** Vegetables
- **F** Fruits
- **C** Carbohydrates
- **PD** Protein/Dairy
- **Ft** Fats
- **S** Sweets

Sweets — 75 calories a day or 525 calories a week
→ Write in your calories here.

Fats

Protein/Dairy

Carbohydrates

Fruits

Vegetables

**WHAT I ATE TODAY FROM THE PYRAMID:**
Check off the circles in the food group servings above as you record food and beverage items in the table at left. For sweets, give your best estimate of the total number of calories for the day.

**TODAY'S DATE:**

**TODAY'S GOAL:**

**NOTES ABOUT TODAY:**
It's weigh-in day ~ record my weight in the weekly Review and the Weight Record.

**WHAT I ATE TODAY:**

Number of servings per food group

| ⏱ Time | Food item | Amount | V | F | C | PD | Ft | S |
|--------|-----------|--------|---|---|---|----|----|---|
| | | | | | | | | |
| | | | | | | | | |
| | | | | | | | | |
| | | | | | | | | |
| | | | | | | | | |
| | | | | | | | | |
| | | | | | | | | |
| | | | | | | | | |
| | | | | | | | | |
| | | | | | | | | |
| | | | | | | | | |
| | | | | | | | | |

**TODAY'S ACTIVITIES:**

🕐 Time

| | |
|---|---|
| | |
| | |
| | |
| Total time (in minutes) | |

**REMINDER:**
Record your weight for today in the weekly Review and the Weight Record.

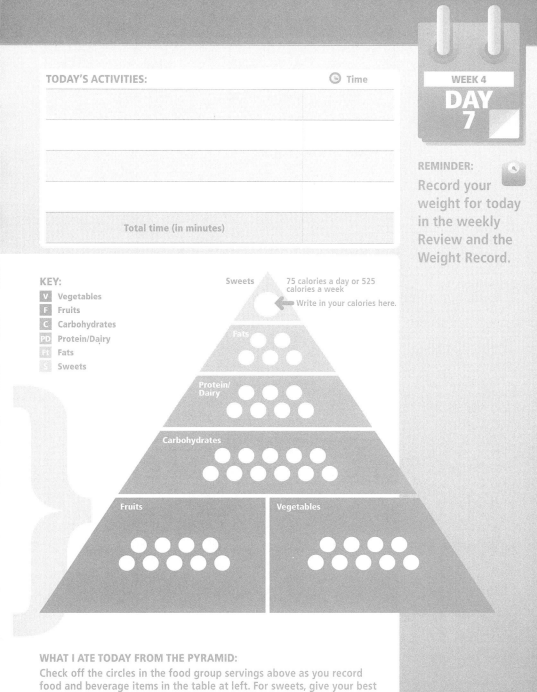

**KEY:**
- **V** Vegetables
- **F** Fruits
- **C** Carbohydrates
- **PD** Protein/Dairy
- **Ft** Fats
- **S** Sweets

**Sweets**
75 calories a day or 525 calories a week

← Write in your calories here.

**Fats**

**Protein/ Dairy**

**Carbohydrates**

**Fruits**

**Vegetables**

**WHAT I ATE TODAY FROM THE PYRAMID:**
Check off the circles in the food group servings above as you record food and beverage items in the table at left. For sweets, give your best estimate of the total number of calories for the day.

| My start weight | | I FEEL: | I'M MOST PROUD OF: |
|---|---|---|---|
| Minus my weight today | | ○ Terrific | |
| | | ○ Good | |
| = Equals my weight change | | ○ So-so | |
| | | ○ Discouraged | |
| | | ○ Like giving up | |

**WHAT WORKED WELL:**

**WHAT DIDN'T WORK AS WELL:**

## DID I REACH MY SERVINGS GOALS FOR THIS WEEK?

| Food group | Daily servings | Day 1 | Day 2 | Day 3 | Day 4 | Day 5 | Day 6 | Day 7 |
|---|---|---|---|---|---|---|---|---|
| Vegetables | | ○ | ○ | ○ | ○ | ○ | ○ | ○ |
| Fruits | | ○ | ○ | ○ | ○ | ○ | ○ | ○ |
| Carbohydrates | | ○ | ○ | ○ | ○ | ○ | ○ | ○ |
| Protein/Dairy | | ○ | ○ | ○ | ○ | ○ | ○ | ○ |
| Fats | | ○ | ○ | ○ | ○ | ○ | ○ | ○ |
| Sweets | | ○ | ○ | ○ | ○ | ○ | ○ | ○ |

**DIRECTIONS:**
1. Write your daily serving goals for each food group in the table above.
2. Compare the serving totals that you recorded for each day of the past week with your goals.
3. Check off the circles in the table above if your serving totals have met your goals.

**NEW FOOD I WOULD LIKE TO TRY:**

**NEW WAYS TO ADD ACTIVITY TO MY DAY:**

**REMINDER:** Calculate your weight change in this Review and record it in the Weight Record.

**HOW MANY STEPS A DAY DID I TAKE (IF I USED A PEDOMETER)?**

| Day 1 | Day 2 | Day 3 | Day 4 | Day 5 | Day 6 | Day 7 |
|-------|-------|-------|-------|-------|-------|-------|
|       |       |       |       |       |       |       |

**HOW MANY MINUTES A DAY WAS I ACTIVE?**

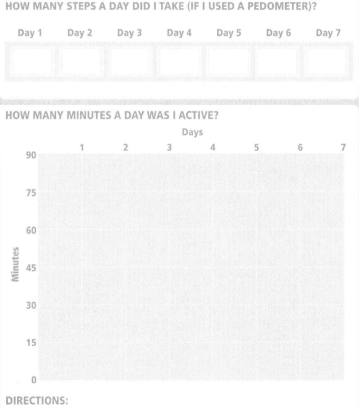

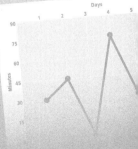

**DIRECTIONS:**
1. Add a dot for your total minutes of activity for each day of last week.
2. Connect each dot on the chart with a line.

See a sample chart to the right. →

The samples above show how you can fill out your servings goals table and your activity chart for your weekly Review.

| Day | Breakfast | Lunch | Dinner | Snack |
|---|---|---|---|---|
| EXAMPLE | cereal banana | spaghetti fruit salad | tuna wrap baby carrots | crackers and cheese |
| 1 | | | | |
| 2 | | | | |
| 3 | | | | |
| 4 | | | | |
| 5 | | | | |
| 6 | | | | |
| 7 | | | | |

| Exercise and activities | Events and special plans |
|---|---|
| swim class @ 11am<br>walk to work | kids ballgame @ 6pm<br>note: supper will be on the go |
|  |  |
|  |  |
|  |  |
|  |  |
|  |  |
|  |  |

**USING THE PLANNER:**
Organize your plans for meals, activities and exercise in the coming week. Note upcoming events that may affect your weight program, such as travel, eating out, social occasions and vacations.

| MAIN MEAL OR MEALS OF THE DAY | HOW MUCH |
|---|---|
|  |  |

EASY AS 1, 2, 3:

This page allows you to check how well a meal meets your recommended servings goals.

1. Write down what you're planning to eat for this meal (or for the entire day).
2. Calculate the number of servings based on how much you're planning to eat.
3. Be sure to include the food items from your menu in your Shopping List.

## PYRAMID SERVINGS FOR THIS MEAL

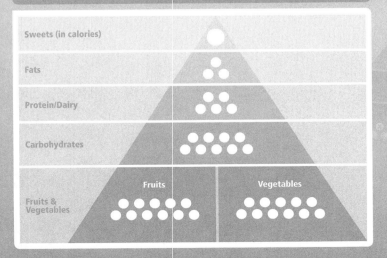

Sweets (in calories)

Fats

Protein/Dairy

Carbohydrates

Fruits & Vegetables — Fruits — Vegetables

◄ Check off the number of servings on the pyramid at left.

WEEK 5 PLANNER

# MEAL PLANNER

| MAIN MEAL OR MEALS OF THE DAY | HOW MUCH |
|---|---|
|  |  |

EASY AS 1, 2, 3:

This page allows you to check how well a meal meets your recommended servings goals.

1. Write down what you're planning to eat for this meal (or for the entire day).
2. Calculate the number of servings based on how much you're planning to eat.
3. Be sure to include the food items from your menu in your Shopping List.

## PYRAMID SERVINGS FOR THIS MEAL

| | |
|---|---|
| Sweets (in calories) | ○ |
| Fats | ○ ○ ○ |
| Protein/Dairy | ○ ○ ○ ○ ○ |
| Carbohydrates | ○ ○ ○ ○ ○ ○ ○ |

| Fruits | Vegetables |
|---|---|
| ○ ○ ○ ○ ○ ○ ○ ○ ○ ○ | ○ ○ ○ ○ ○ ○ ○ ○ ○ ○ |

Fruits & Vegetables

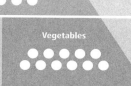

◄ Check off the number of servings on the pyramid at left.

## MENU FOR THE DAY

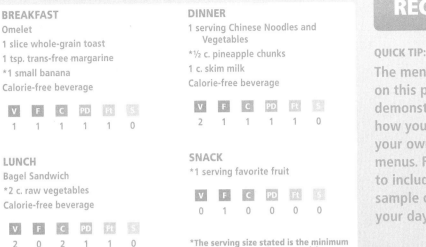

**BREAKFAST**
Omelet
1 slice whole-grain toast
1 tsp. trans-free margarine
*1 small banana
Calorie-free beverage

| V | F | C | PD | Ft | S |
|---|---|---|----|----|---|
| 1 | 1 | 1 | 1  | 1  | 0 |

**DINNER**
1 serving Chinese Noodles and Vegetables
*½ c. pineapple chunks
1 c. skim milk
Calorie-free beverage

| V | F | C | PD | Ft | S |
|---|---|---|----|----|---|
| 2 | 1 | 1 | 1  | 1  | 0 |

**LUNCH**
Bagel Sandwich
*2 c. raw vegetables
Calorie-free beverage

| V | F | C | PD | Ft | S |
|---|---|---|----|----|---|
| 2 | 0 | 2 | 1  | 1  | 0 |

**SNACK**
*1 serving favorite fruit

| V | F | C | PD | Ft | S |
|---|---|---|----|----|---|
| 0 | 1 | 0 | 0  | 0  | 0 |

*The serving size stated is the minimum amount. Eat as much as you wish.

**QUICK TIP:**
The menu on this page demonstrates how you can plan your own daily menus. Feel free to include this sample on one of your days.

## BREAKFAST RECIPE

### Omelet

- Mix ½ cup egg substitute with ½ cup diced onions, tomatoes, green peppers and mushrooms, and cook until set.

## LUNCH RECIPE

### Bagel Sandwich

- Spread 1 whole-grain bagel with 1 tablespoon reduced-calorie mayonnaise. Top with 2 ounces lean ham, lettuce, tomato and onion slice.

## DINNER RECIPE

### Chinese Noodles and Vegetables

- Prepare 1 package ramen noodles as directed. Rinse and set aside. Sauté 1 tablespoon grated ginger and 1 tablespoon chopped garlic in 1 tablespoon sesame oil and 1 tablespoon peanut oil. Add ½ cup broccoli florets and sauté 3 minutes. Add ½ cup of each: bean sprouts, fresh spinach and cherry tomato halves. Add noodles and toss. Sprinkle with chopped green onions and soy sauce.

| Fresh produce | Whole grains | Meat & dairy |
| --- | --- | --- |
| | | |

| Frozen goods | Canned goods | Miscellaneous |
| --- | --- | --- |
| | | |

QUICK TIP:

Create your shopping list for the week before going to the grocery store. You'll have all the ingredients on hand at the time you prepare a meal.

| Fresh produce | Whole grains |
| --- | --- |
| 10 large tomatoes | 8 oz package spaghetti |
| 2 red peppers | 1 loaf rye bread |
| summer squash | 1 package eng muffins |
| zucchini | |
| 1 bag baby carrots | bag of pita |
| cherries | |
| 3 grapefruit | |

Add to your Shopping List as you plan your menus for the week.

**TODAY'S DATE:**

**TODAY'S GOAL:**

**NOTES ABOUT TODAY:**

**WHAT I ATE TODAY:**

Number of servings per food group

| Time | Food item | Amount | V | F | C | PD | Ft | S |
|------|-----------|--------|---|---|---|----|----|---|
|      |           |        |   |   |   |    |    |   |
|      |           |        |   |   |   |    |    |   |
|      |           |        |   |   |   |    |    |   |
|      |           |        |   |   |   |    |    |   |
|      |           |        |   |   |   |    |    |   |
|      |           |        |   |   |   |    |    |   |
|      |           |        |   |   |   |    |    |   |
|      |           |        |   |   |   |    |    |   |
|      |           |        |   |   |   |    |    |   |
|      |           |        |   |   |   |    |    |   |
|      |           |        |   |   |   |    |    |   |
|      |           |        |   |   |   |    |    |   |

**TODAY'S ACTIVITIES:**                                      🕐 **Time**

|  |  |
|---|---|
|  |  |
|  |  |
|  |  |
| **Total time (in minutes)** |  |

**MOTIVATION TIP:**
Make sure you're not skipping breakfast by keeping food handy that you can carry with you in the morning. Eat in the car, on the train or bus, or at work.

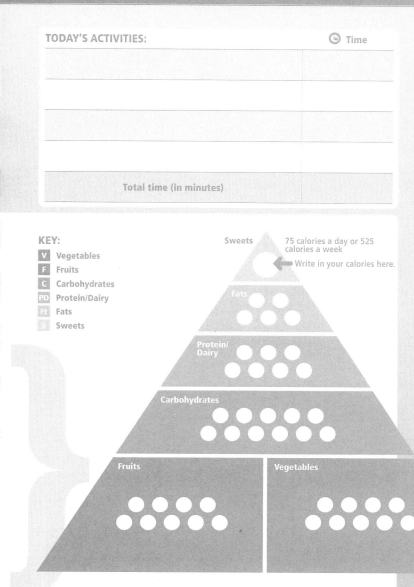

**KEY:**
- V  Vegetables
- F  Fruits
- C  Carbohydrates
- PD Protein/Dairy
- Ft Fats
- S  Sweets

Sweets — 75 calories a day or 525 calories a week
← Write in your calories here.

Fats

Protein/Dairy

Carbohydrates

Fruits        Vegetables

**WHAT I ATE TODAY FROM THE PYRAMID:**
Check off the circles in the food group servings above as you record food and beverage items in the table at left. For sweets, give your best estimate of the total number of calories for the day.

**TODAY'S DATE:**

**TODAY'S GOAL:**

**NOTES ABOUT TODAY:**

**WHAT I ATE TODAY:**

Number of servings per food group

| Time | Food item | Amount | V | F | C | PD | PK | S |
|------|-----------|--------|---|---|---|----|----|----|
|  |  |  |  |  |  |  |  |  |
|  |  |  |  |  |  |  |  |  |
|  |  |  |  |  |  |  |  |  |
|  |  |  |  |  |  |  |  |  |
|  |  |  |  |  |  |  |  |  |
|  |  |  |  |  |  |  |  |  |
|  |  |  |  |  |  |  |  |  |
|  |  |  |  |  |  |  |  |  |
|  |  |  |  |  |  |  |  |  |
|  |  |  |  |  |  |  |  |  |
|  |  |  |  |  |  |  |  |  |
|  |  |  |  |  |  |  |  |  |

**TODAY'S ACTIVITIES:**　　　　　　　　　　　🕐 Time

Total time (in minutes)

**MOTIVATION TIP:**
Every bit of food you eat doesn't have to be an excellent source of nutrition. Your main goal is to choose foods that promote good health more often than you choose those that don't.

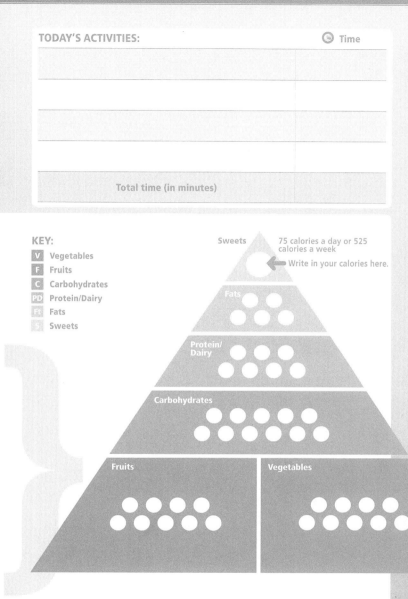

**KEY:**

- **V.** Vegetables
- **F.** Fruits
- **C.** Carbohydrates
- **PD.** Protein/Dairy
- **Ft.** Fats
- **S.** Sweets

Sweets　　75 calories a day or 525 calories a week
← Write in your calories here.

Fats

Protein/Dairy

Carbohydrates

Fruits　　　　　Vegetables

**WHAT I ATE TODAY FROM THE PYRAMID:**
Check off the circles in the food group servings above as you record food and beverage items in the table at left. For sweets, give your best estimate of the total number of calories for the day.

**TODAY'S DATE:**

**TODAY'S GOAL:**

**NOTES ABOUT TODAY:**

**WHAT I ATE TODAY:**

Number of servings per food group

| Time | Food item | Amount | V | F | C | PD | Ft | S |
|------|-----------|--------|---|---|---|----|----|----|
|      |           |        |   |   |   |    |    |    |
|      |           |        |   |   |   |    |    |    |
|      |           |        |   |   |   |    |    |    |
|      |           |        |   |   |   |    |    |    |
|      |           |        |   |   |   |    |    |    |
|      |           |        |   |   |   |    |    |    |
|      |           |        |   |   |   |    |    |    |
|      |           |        |   |   |   |    |    |    |
|      |           |        |   |   |   |    |    |    |
|      |           |        |   |   |   |    |    |    |
|      |           |        |   |   |   |    |    |    |

**TODAY'S ACTIVITIES:**     🕐 Time

Total time (in minutes)

**MOTIVATION TIP:**
Make exercise a priority today. If you treat it as secondary, exercise will quickly drop to the bottom of your to-do list.

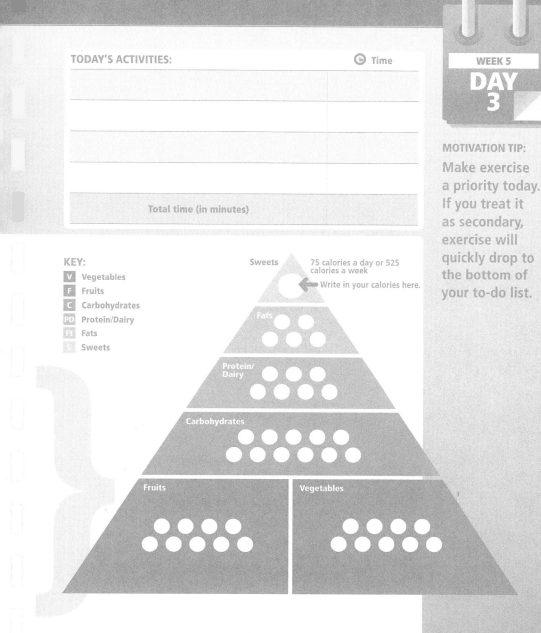

**KEY:**
- **V** Vegetables
- **F** Fruits
- **C** Carbohydrates
- **PD** Protein/Dairy
- **Ft** Fats
- **S** Sweets

Sweets    75 calories a day or 525 calories a week

Write in your calories here.

Fats

Protein/Dairy

Carbohydrates

Fruits

Vegetables

## WHAT I ATE TODAY FROM THE PYRAMID:

Check off the circles in the food group servings above as you record food and beverage items in the table at left. For sweets, give your best estimate of the total number of calories for the day.

**TODAY'S DATE:**

**TODAY'S GOAL:**

**NOTES ABOUT TODAY:**

**WHAT I ATE TODAY:**

Number of servings per food group

| Time | Food item | Amount | V | F | C | PD | Ft | S |
|------|-----------|--------|---|---|---|----|----|---|
|      |           |        |   |   |   |    |    |   |
|      |           |        |   |   |   |    |    |   |
|      |           |        |   |   |   |    |    |   |
|      |           |        |   |   |   |    |    |   |
|      |           |        |   |   |   |    |    |   |
|      |           |        |   |   |   |    |    |   |
|      |           |        |   |   |   |    |    |   |
|      |           |        |   |   |   |    |    |   |
|      |           |        |   |   |   |    |    |   |
|      |           |        |   |   |   |    |    |   |
|      |           |        |   |   |   |    |    |   |
|      |           |        |   |   |   |    |    |   |

**TODAY'S ACTIVITIES:**

🕐 Time

|  |  |
|---|---|
|  |  |
|  |  |
|  |  |
| Total time (in minutes) |  |

**MOTIVATION TIP:**
Exercise should not be painful. Muscle soreness after exercise is common, but pain during exercise can be a signal of impending injury. Stop what you're doing and consult your doctor.

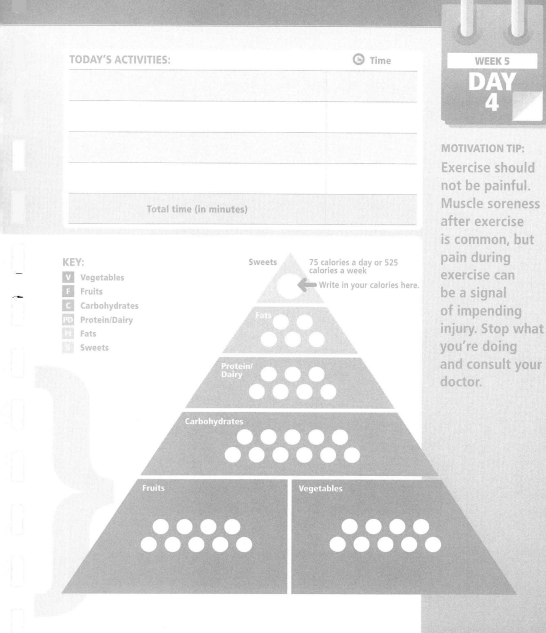

**KEY:**
- V  Vegetables
- F  Fruits
- C  Carbohydrates
- PD  Protein/Dairy
- H  Fats
- S  Sweets

Sweets

75 calories a day or 525 calories a week

Write in your calories here.

Fats

Protein/Dairy

Carbohydrates

Fruits

Vegetables

**WHAT I ATE TODAY FROM THE PYRAMID:**
Check off the circles in the food group servings above as you record food and beverage items in the table at left. For sweets, give your best estimate of the total number of calories for the day.

**TODAY'S DATE:**

**TODAY'S GOAL:**

**NOTES ABOUT TODAY:**

**WHAT I ATE TODAY:**

Number of servings per food group

| ⏱ Time | Food item | Amount | V | F | C | PD | Ft | S |
|--------|-----------|--------|---|---|---|----|----|----|
|        |           |        |   |   |   |    |    |   |
|        |           |        |   |   |   |    |    |   |
|        |           |        |   |   |   |    |    |   |
|        |           |        |   |   |   |    |    |   |
|        |           |        |   |   |   |    |    |   |
|        |           |        |   |   |   |    |    |   |
|        |           |        |   |   |   |    |    |   |
|        |           |        |   |   |   |    |    |   |
|        |           |        |   |   |   |    |    |   |
|        |           |        |   |   |   |    |    |   |
|        |           |        |   |   |   |    |    |   |
|        |           |        |   |   |   |    |    |   |

## TODAY'S ACTIVITIES:

🕐 Time

_____

_____

_____

_____

Total time (in minutes)

**MOTIVATION TIP:**
Eating to ease stress almost always ends in overeating. Look for other ways to cope with stress, including exercise, regular mealtimes and getting enough sleep.

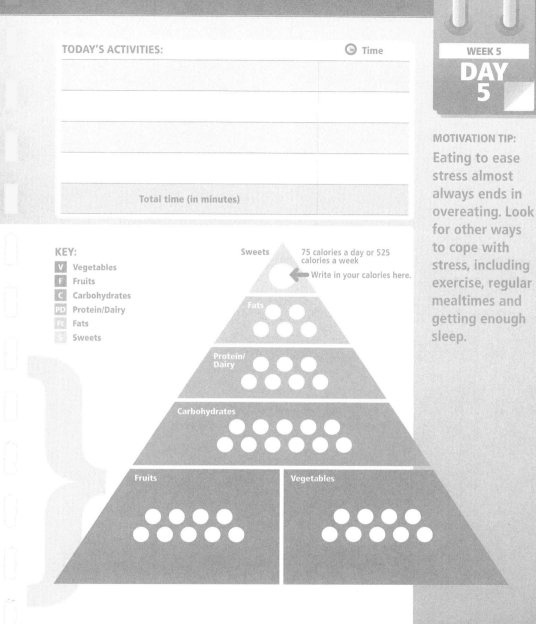

**KEY:**

- **V** Vegetables
- **F** Fruits
- **C** Carbohydrates
- **PD** Protein/Dairy
- **F** Fats
- **S** Sweets

Sweets

75 calories a day or 525 calories a week

← Write in your calories here.

Fats

Protein/Dairy

Carbohydrates

Fruits

Vegetables

## WHAT I ATE TODAY FROM THE PYRAMID:

Check off the circles in the food group servings above as you record food and beverage items in the table at left. For sweets, give your best estimate of the total number of calories for the day.

**TODAY'S DATE:**

**TODAY'S GOAL:**

**NOTES ABOUT TODAY:**

**WHAT I ATE TODAY:**

Number of servings per food group

| Time | Food item | Amount | V | F | C | PD | Ft | S |
|------|-----------|--------|---|---|---|----|----|----|
|  |  |  |  |  |  |  |  |  |
|  |  |  |  |  |  |  |  |  |
|  |  |  |  |  |  |  |  |  |
|  |  |  |  |  |  |  |  |  |
|  |  |  |  |  |  |  |  |  |
|  |  |  |  |  |  |  |  |  |
|  |  |  |  |  |  |  |  |  |
|  |  |  |  |  |  |  |  |  |
|  |  |  |  |  |  |  |  |  |
|  |  |  |  |  |  |  |  |  |

## TODAY'S ACTIVITIES:

🕐 Time

_____

_____

_____

_____

**Total time (in minutes)**

**MOTIVATION TIP:**

Keep your response to an eating or exercise lapse simple. Focus on the things you know you can do and avoid drastic changes. You'll soon get back on track.

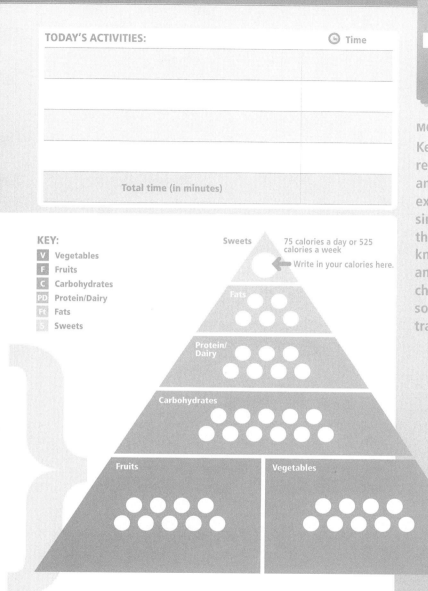

**KEY:**

- **V** Vegetables
- **F** Fruits
- **C** Carbohydrates
- **PD** Protein/Dairy
- **Ft** Fats
- **S** Sweets

Sweets

75 calories a day or 525 calories a week

Write in your calories here.

Fats

Protein/Dairy

Carbohydrates

Fruits

Vegetables

**WHAT I ATE TODAY FROM THE PYRAMID:**

Check off the circles in the food group servings above as you record food and beverage items in the table at left. For sweets, give your best estimate of the total number of calories for the day.

**TODAY'S DATE:**

**TODAY'S GOAL:**

**NOTES ABOUT TODAY:**
It's weigh-in day ~ record my weight in the weekly Review and the Weight Record.

**WHAT I ATE TODAY:**

| Time | Food item | Amount | V | F | C | PD | Ft | S |
|------|-----------|--------|---|---|---|----|----|---|
| | | | | | | | | |
| | | | | | | | | |
| | | | | | | | | |
| | | | | | | | | |
| | | | | | | | | |
| | | | | | | | | |
| | | | | | | | | |
| | | | | | | | | |
| | | | | | | | | |
| | | | | | | | | |
| | | | | | | | | |
| | | | | | | | | |
| | | | | | | | | |
| | | | | | | | | |

Number of servings per food group

**TODAY'S ACTIVITIES:**

🕐 Time

Total time (in minutes)

**REMINDER:** 🔧

Record your weight for today in the weekly Review and the Weight Record.

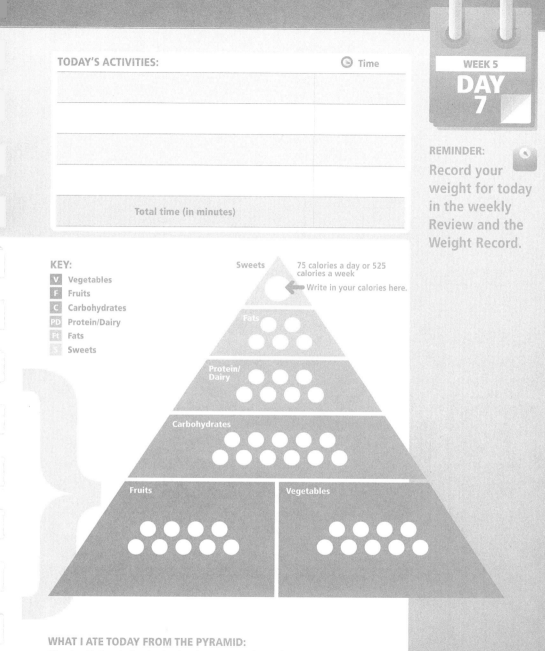

**KEY:**

- **V** Vegetables
- **F** Fruits
- **C** Carbohydrates
- **PD** Protein/Dairy
- **Ft** Fats
- **S** Sweets

Sweets — 75 calories a day or 525 calories a week

Write in your calories here.

Fats

Protein/Dairy

Carbohydrates

Fruits

Vegetables

**WHAT I ATE TODAY FROM THE PYRAMID:**

Check off the circles in the food group servings above as you record food and beverage items in the table at left. For sweets, give your best estimate of the total number of calories for the day.

My start weight:

Minus my weight today:

= Equals my weight change:

**I FEEL:**
- Terrific
- Good
- So-so
- Discouraged
- Like giving up

**I'M MOST PROUD OF:**

**WHAT WORKED WELL:**

**WHAT DIDN'T WORK AS WELL:**

**DID I REACH MY SERVINGS GOALS FOR THIS WEEK?**

| Food group | Daily servings | Day 1 | Day 2 | Day 3 | Day 4 | Day 5 | Day 6 | Day 7 |
|---|---|---|---|---|---|---|---|---|
| Vegetables | | | | | | | | |
| Fruits | | | | | | | | |
| Carbohydrates | | | | | | | | |
| Protein/Dairy | | | | | | | | |
| Fats | | | | | | | | |
| Sweets | | | | | | | | |

**DIRECTIONS:**
1. Write your daily serving goals for each food group in the table above.
2. Compare the serving totals that you recorded for each day of the past week with your goals.
3. Check off the circles in the table above if your serving totals have met your goals.

**NEW FOOD I WOULD LIKE TO TRY:**

**NEW WAYS TO ADD ACTIVITY TO MY DAY:**

**REMINDER:**
Calculate your weight change in this Review and record it in the Weight Record.

**HOW MANY STEPS A DAY DID I TAKE (IF I USED A PEDOMETER)?**

| Day 1 | Day 2 | Day 3 | Day 4 | Day 5 | Day 6 | Day 7 |
|-------|-------|-------|-------|-------|-------|-------|
|       |       |       |       |       |       |       |

**HOW MANY MINUTES A DAY WAS I ACTIVE?**

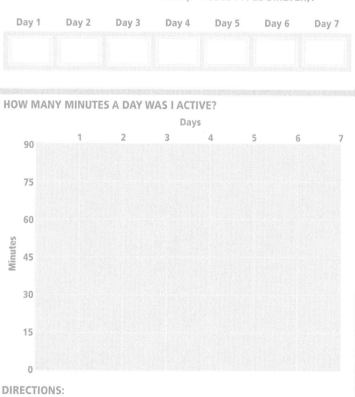

**DIRECTIONS:**
1. Add a dot for your total minutes of activity for each day of last week.
2. Connect each dot on the chart with a line.

See a sample chart to the right. →

The samples above show how you can fill out your servings goals table and your activity chart for your weekly Review.

| Day | Breakfast | Lunch | Dinner | Snack |
|---|---|---|---|---|
| EXAMPLE | cereal<br>banana | spaghetti<br>fruit salad | tuna wrap<br>baby carrots | crackers<br>and cheese |
| 1 | | | | |
| 2 | | | | |
| 3 | | | | |
| 4 | | | | |
| 5 | | | | |
| 6 | | | | |
| 7 | | | | |

| Exercise and activities | Events and special plans |
|---|---|
| swim class @ 11am<br>walk to work | kids ballgame @ 6pm<br>note: supper will be on the go |
| | |
| | |
| | |
| | |
| | |
| | |
| | |

# WEEK AT A GLANCE

**USING THE PLANNER:**

Organize your plans for meals, activities and exercise in the coming week. Note upcoming events that may affect your weight program, such as travel, eating out, social occasions and vacations.

| MAIN MEAL OR MEALS OF THE DAY | HOW MUCH |
|---|---|
| | |

**EASY AS 1, 2, 3:**

This page allows you to check how well a meal meets your recommended servings goals.

1. Write down what you're planning to eat for this meal (or for the entire day).
2. Calculate the number of servings based on how much you're planning to eat.
3. Be sure to include the food items from your menu in your Shopping List.

## PYRAMID SERVINGS FOR THIS MEAL

| | |
|---|---|
| Sweets (in calories) | |
| Fats | |
| Protein/Dairy | |
| Carbohydrates | |
| Fruits & Vegetables | Fruits / Vegetables |

◄ Check off the number of servings on the pyramid at left.

75

WEEK 6 PLANNER
# MEAL PLANNER

| MAIN MEAL OR MEALS OF THE DAY | HOW MUCH |
|---|---|
| | |

## EASY AS 1, 2, 3:

This page allows you to check how well a meal meets your recommended servings goals.

1. Write down what you're planning to eat for this meal (or for the entire day).

2. Calculate the number of servings based on how much you're planning to eat.

3. Be sure to include the food items from your menu in your Shopping List.

## PYRAMID SERVINGS FOR THIS MEAL

| | |
|---|---|
| Sweets (in calories) | ○ |
| Fats | ○○○ |
| Protein/Dairy | ○○○○○ |
| Carbohydrates | ○○○○○○○ |

| Fruits | Vegetables |
|---|---|
| ○○○○○○○ | ○○○○○○ |

Fruits & Vegetables

◄ Check off the number of servings on the pyramid at left.

## MENU FOR THE DAY

### BREAKFAST
2 small muffins, any flavor
2 tsp. trans-free margarine
*2 pear halves
Calorie-free beverage

| V | F | C | PD | Ft | S |
|---|---|---|----|----|----|
| 0 | 1 | 2 | 0 | 2 | 0 |

### LUNCH
Chicken wrap
*1 medium tomato
*1 medium apple
Calorie-free beverage

| V | F | C | PD | Ft | S |
|---|---|---|----|----|----|
| 1 | 1 | 1 | 1 | 1 | 0 |

### DINNER
4 oz. lean pork, grilled or broiled
⅓ c. cooked brown rice
1 serving Sesame Asparagus and
   Carrot Stir-Fry
1 small slice angel food cake
*1 c. berries
Calorie-free beverage

| V | F | C | PD | Ft | S |
|---|---|---|----|----|----|
| 2 | 1 | 1 | 2 | 1 | 0 |

### SNACK
*1 serving favorite vegetable

| V | F | C | PD | Ft | S |
|---|---|---|----|----|----|
| 1 | 0 | 0 | 0 | 0 | 0 |

*The serving size stated is the minimum amount. Eat as much as you wish.

QUICK TIP:

The menu on this page demonstrates how you can plan your own daily menus. Feel free to include this sample on one of your days.

## DINNER RECIPE

### Sesame Asparagus and Carrot Stir-Fry

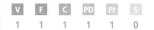

24 asparagus stalks
6   large carrots
¼   C. water
1   tbsp. grated fresh ginger
1   tbsp. reduced-sodium soy sauce
1½ tsp. sesame oil
1½ tbsp. sesame seeds, toasted

■ Cut the asparagus into ½-inch-thick slices. Cut the carrots into ¼-inch-thick slices.

■ Coat a wok or frying pan with cooking spray and place over high heat. Add the carrots and stir-fry for 4 minutes. Add the asparagus and water. Stir and toss to combine. Cover and cook until the vegetables are barely tender, about 2 minutes. Uncover and add the ginger. Stir-fry until remaining water evaporates, about 1 to 2 minutes.

■ Add the soy sauce, sesame oil and sesame seeds. Stir-fry to coat the vegetables evenly. Dish onto individual plates and serve.

| Fresh produce | Whole grains | Meat & dairy |
|---|---|---|
| | | |

| Frozen goods | Canned goods | Miscellaneous |
|---|---|---|
| | | |

**QUICK TIP:**

Create your shopping list for the week before going to the grocery store. You'll have all the ingredients on hand at the time you prepare a meal.

| Fresh produce | Whole grain |
|---|---|
| 10 large tomatoes | 8 oz package spaghetti |
| 2 red peppers | 1 loaf rye bre |
| summer squash | 1 package e muffins |
| zucchini | |
| 1 bag baby carrots | bag of pita |
| cherries | |
| 3 grapefruit | |

Add to your Shopping List as you plan your menus for the week.

**TODAY'S DATE:**

**TODAY'S GOAL:**

**NOTES ABOUT TODAY:**

**WHAT I ATE TODAY:**                                    **Number of servings per food group**

| Time | Food item | Amount | V | F | C | PD | Ft | S |
|------|-----------|--------|---|---|---|----|----|----|
|      |           |        |   |   |   |    |    |   |
|      |           |        |   |   |   |    |    |   |
|      |           |        |   |   |   |    |    |   |
|      |           |        |   |   |   |    |    |   |
|      |           |        |   |   |   |    |    |   |
|      |           |        |   |   |   |    |    |   |
|      |           |        |   |   |   |    |    |   |
|      |           |        |   |   |   |    |    |   |
|      |           |        |   |   |   |    |    |   |
|      |           |        |   |   |   |    |    |   |
|      |           |        |   |   |   |    |    |   |

## TODAY'S ACTIVITIES:

🕐 Time

|  |  |
|---|---|
|  |  |
|  |  |
|  |  |
|  |  |
| **Total time (in minutes)** |  |

**MOTIVATION TIP:**
Try listening to music while you exercise. Upbeat music can rev you up. It makes the workout seem easier and the time pass more quickly.

**KEY:**
- **V** Vegetables
- **F** Fruits
- **C** Carbohydrates
- **PD** Protein/Dairy
- **FL** Fats
- **S** Sweets

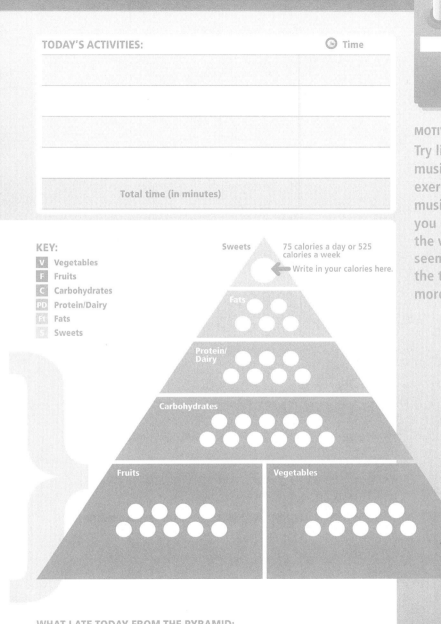

Sweets — 75 calories a day or 525 calories a week
← Write in your calories here.

Fats

Protein/Dairy

Carbohydrates

Fruits            Vegetables

**WHAT I ATE TODAY FROM THE PYRAMID:**
Check off the circles in the food group servings above as you record food and beverage items in the table at left. For sweets, give your best estimate of the total number of calories for the day.

**TODAY'S DATE:**

**TODAY'S GOAL:**

**NOTES ABOUT TODAY:**

**WHAT I ATE TODAY:**                              Number of servings per food group

| Time | Food item | Amount | V | F | C | PD | Pr | S |
|------|-----------|--------|---|---|---|----|----|----|
|      |           |        |   |   |   |    |    |    |
|      |           |        |   |   |   |    |    |    |
|      |           |        |   |   |   |    |    |    |
|      |           |        |   |   |   |    |    |    |
|      |           |        |   |   |   |    |    |    |
|      |           |        |   |   |   |    |    |    |
|      |           |        |   |   |   |    |    |    |
|      |           |        |   |   |   |    |    |    |
|      |           |        |   |   |   |    |    |    |
|      |           |        |   |   |   |    |    |    |
|      |           |        |   |   |   |    |    |    |
|      |           |        |   |   |   |    |    |    |
|      |           |        |   |   |   |    |    |    |
|      |           |        |   |   |   |    |    |    |

**TODAY'S ACTIVITIES:**

🕐 Time

| | |
|---|---|
| | |
| | |
| | |
| | |
| Total time (in minutes) | |

**MOTIVATION TIP:**
Don't shop on an empty stomach. Eat something before you go to the store. If you're hungry, it's harder to resist the bright packaging and enticing smells of many high-calorie foods.

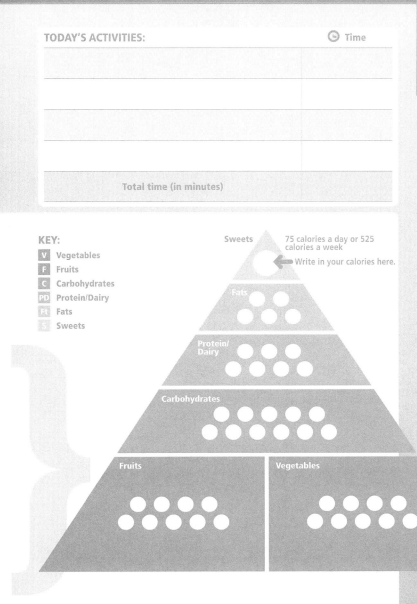

**KEY:**
- **V** Vegetables
- **F** Fruits
- **C** Carbohydrates
- **PD** Protein/Dairy
- **Ft** Fats
- **S** Sweets

Sweets — 75 calories a day or 525 calories a week

← Write in your calories here.

Fats

Protein/Dairy

Carbohydrates

Fruits

Vegetables

**WHAT I ATE TODAY FROM THE PYRAMID:**
Check off the circles in the food group servings above as you record food and beverage items in the table at left. For sweets, give your best estimate of the total number of calories for the day.

**TODAY'S DATE:**

**TODAY'S GOAL:**

**NOTES ABOUT TODAY:**

**WHAT I ATE TODAY:**

Number of servings per food group

| 🕐 Time | Food item | Amount | V | F | C | PD | Ft | S |
|---------|-----------|--------|---|---|---|----|----|----|
| | | | | | | | | |
| | | | | | | | | |
| | | | | | | | | |
| | | | | | | | | |
| | | | | | | | | |
| | | | | | | | | |
| | | | | | | | | |
| | | | | | | | | |
| | | | | | | | | |
| | | | | | | | | |
| | | | | | | | | |
| | | | | | | | | |

**TODAY'S ACTIVITIES:**

🕐 Time

Total time (in minutes)

**MOTIVATION TIP:**
Acknowledge that you're a person of value who can contribute to your community and to others, regardless of what you weigh.

**KEY:**
- **V** Vegetables
- **F** Fruits
- **C** Carbohydrates
- **PD** Protein/Dairy
- **Ft** Fats
- **S** Sweets

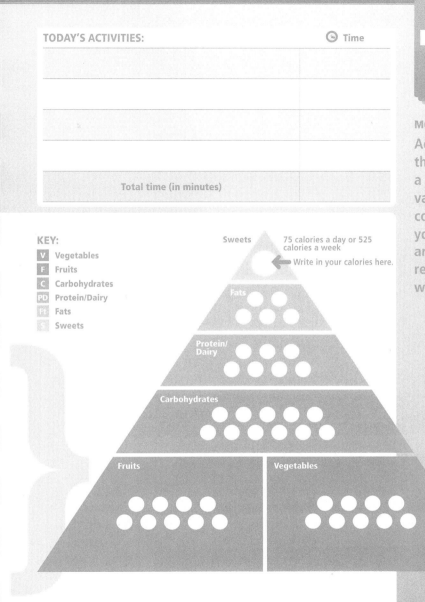

Sweets — 75 calories a day or 525 calories a week
← Write in your calories here.

Fats

Protein/Dairy

Carbohydrates

Fruits

Vegetables

## WHAT I ATE TODAY FROM THE PYRAMID:

Check off the circles in the food group servings above as you record food and beverage items in the table at left. For sweets, give your best estimate of the total number of calories for the day.

**TODAY'S DATE:**

**TODAY'S GOAL:**

**NOTES ABOUT TODAY:**

**WHAT I ATE TODAY:**                                         **Number of servings per food group**

| Time | Food item | Amount | V | F | C | PD | Ft | S |
|------|-----------|--------|---|---|---|----|----|---|
|      |           |        |   |   |   |    |    |   |
|      |           |        |   |   |   |    |    |   |
|      |           |        |   |   |   |    |    |   |
|      |           |        |   |   |   |    |    |   |
|      |           |        |   |   |   |    |    |   |
|      |           |        |   |   |   |    |    |   |
|      |           |        |   |   |   |    |    |   |
|      |           |        |   |   |   |    |    |   |

**TODAY'S ACTIVITIES:**

🕐 Time

Total time (in minutes)

**MOTIVATION TIP:**

Feeling good about what you achieve — even if it seems minor — can help keep you motivated. Each time a goal is met, set a new and more challenging one.

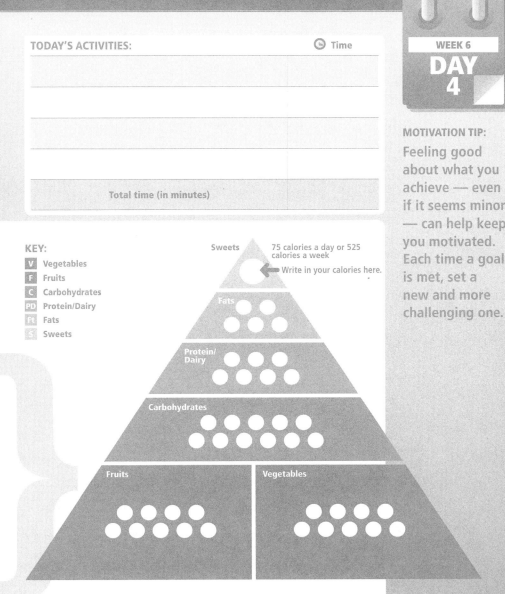

**KEY:**

| | |
|---|---|
| **V** | Vegetables |
| **F** | Fruits |
| **C** | Carbohydrates |
| **PD** | Protein/Dairy |
| **Ft** | Fats |
| **S** | Sweets |

Sweets

75 calories a day or 525 calories a week

← Write in your calories here.

Fats

Protein/Dairy

Carbohydrates

Fruits

Vegetables

**WHAT I ATE TODAY FROM THE PYRAMID:**

Check off the circles in the food group servings above as you record food and beverage items in the table at left. For sweets, give your best estimate of the total number of calories for the day.

**TODAY'S DATE:**

**TODAY'S GOAL:**

**NOTES ABOUT TODAY:**

**WHAT I ATE TODAY:**      Number of servings per food group

| Time | Food item | Amount | V | F | C | PD | Ft | S |
|------|-----------|--------|---|---|---|----|----|----|
|  |  |  |  |  |  |  |  |  |
|  |  |  |  |  |  |  |  |  |
|  |  |  |  |  |  |  |  |  |
|  |  |  |  |  |  |  |  |  |
|  |  |  |  |  |  |  |  |  |
|  |  |  |  |  |  |  |  |  |
|  |  |  |  |  |  |  |  |  |
|  |  |  |  |  |  |  |  |  |
|  |  |  |  |  |  |  |  |  |
|  |  |  |  |  |  |  |  |  |
|  |  |  |  |  |  |  |  |  |
|  |  |  |  |  |  |  |  |  |

**TODAY'S ACTIVITIES:**

🕐 **Time**

_____

_____

_____

_____

| Total time (in minutes) | |
|---|---|

**MOTIVATION TIP:**
Totally denying yourself of a food you enjoy, such as chocolate, is a sure way to fuel a craving. A more sensible approach is to treat yourself to it now and then — but in small amounts.

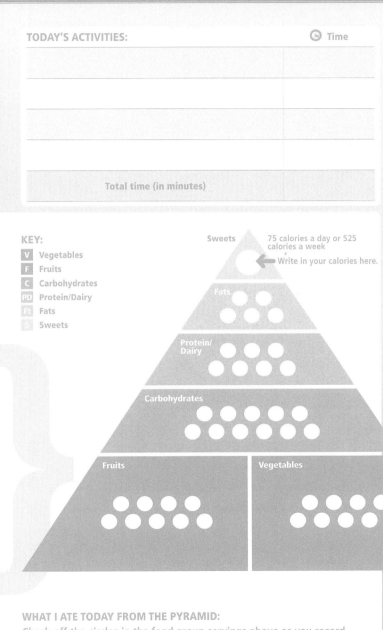

**KEY:**

V  Vegetables
F  Fruits
C  Carbohydrates
PD  Protein/Dairy
FL  Fats
S  Sweets

Sweets  75 calories a day or 525 calories a week
Write in your calories here.

Fats

Protein/Dairy

Carbohydrates

Fruits

Vegetables

**WHAT I ATE TODAY FROM THE PYRAMID:**
Check off the circles in the food group servings above as you record food and beverage items in the table at left. For sweets, give your best estimate of the total number of calories for the day.

**TODAY'S DATE:**

**TODAY'S GOAL:**

**NOTES ABOUT TODAY:**

**WHAT I ATE TODAY:**

Number of servings per food group

| 🕐 Time | Food item | Amount | V | F | C | PD | Ft | S |
|---------|-----------|--------|---|---|---|----|----|---|
| | | | | | | | | |
| | | | | | | | | |
| | | | | | | | | |
| | | | | | | | | |
| | | | | | | | | |
| | | | | | | | | |
| | | | | | | | | |
| | | | | | | | | |
| | | | | | | | | |
| | | | | | | | | |
| | | | | | | | | |
| | | | | | | | | |

**TODAY'S ACTIVITIES:**

🕐 Time

| | |
|---|---|
| | |
| | |
| | |
| Total time (in minutes) | |

**MOTIVATION TIP:**
When you don't have time to make a healthy meal, stop at a grocery store or deli for a healthy sandwich, soup or prepared entreé that's low in fat and calories.

**KEY:**
- **V** Vegetables
- **F** Fruits
- **C** Carbohydrates
- **PD** Protein/Dairy
- **FL** Fats
- **S** Sweets

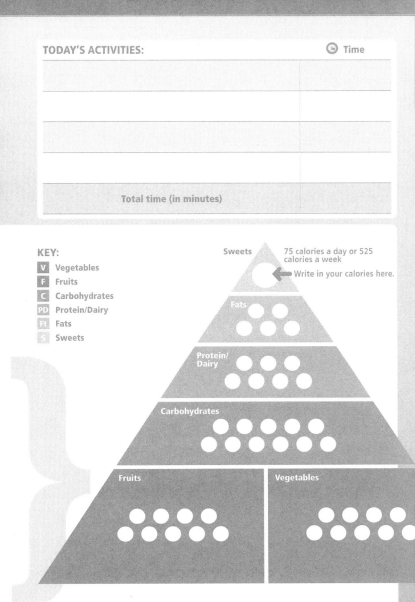

Sweets — 75 calories a day or 525 calories a week
Write in your calories here.

Fats

Protein/Dairy

Carbohydrates

Fruits

Vegetables

**WHAT I ATE TODAY FROM THE PYRAMID:**
Check off the circles in the food group servings above as you record food and beverage items in the table at left. For sweets, give your best estimate of the total number of calories for the day.

**TODAY'S DATE:**

**TODAY'S GOAL:**

**NOTES ABOUT TODAY:**
It's weigh-in day ~ record my weight in the weekly Review and the Weight Record.

**WHAT I ATE TODAY:**

Number of servings per food group

| Time | Food item | Amount | V | F | C | PD | Ft | S |
|------|-----------|--------|---|---|---|----|----|---|
|      |           |        |   |   |   |    |    |   |
|      |           |        |   |   |   |    |    |   |
|      |           |        |   |   |   |    |    |   |
|      |           |        |   |   |   |    |    |   |
|      |           |        |   |   |   |    |    |   |
|      |           |        |   |   |   |    |    |   |
|      |           |        |   |   |   |    |    |   |
|      |           |        |   |   |   |    |    |   |
|      |           |        |   |   |   |    |    |   |
|      |           |        |   |   |   |    |    |   |
|      |           |        |   |   |   |    |    |   |

## TODAY'S ACTIVITIES:

🕐 Time

Total time (in minutes)

REMINDER:
Record your weight for today in the weekly Review and the Weight Record.

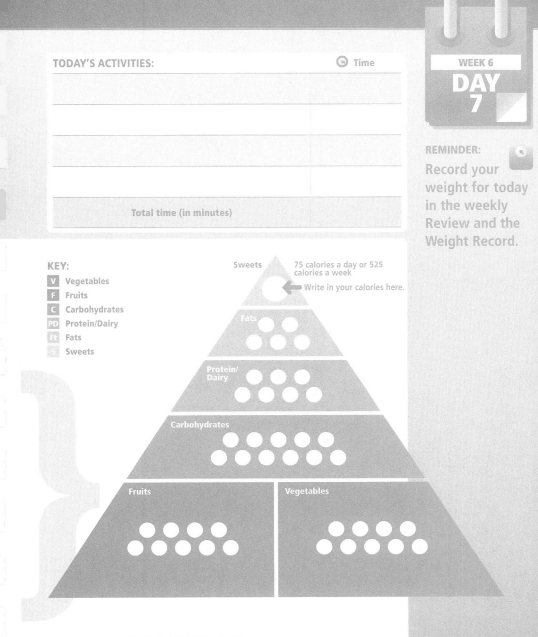

**KEY:**
- **V** Vegetables
- **F** Fruits
- **C** Carbohydrates
- **PD** Protein/Dairy
- **Ft** Fats
- **S** Sweets

Sweets — 75 calories a day or 525 calories a week

Write in your calories here.

Fats

Protein/Dairy

Carbohydrates

Fruits

Vegetables

## WHAT I ATE TODAY FROM THE PYRAMID:

Check off the circles in the food group servings above as you record food and beverage items in the table at left. For sweets, give your best estimate of the total number of calories for the day.

**My start weight**

**Minus my weight today**

**= Equals my weight change**

**I FEEL:**
- Terrific
- Good
- So-so
- Discouraged
- Like giving up

**I'M MOST PROUD OF:**

**WHAT WORKED WELL:**

**WHAT DIDN'T WORK AS WELL:**

**DID I REACH MY SERVINGS GOALS FOR THIS WEEK?**

| Food group | Daily servings | Day 1 | Day 2 | Day 3 | Day 4 | Day 5 | Day 6 | Day 7 |
|---|---|---|---|---|---|---|---|---|
| Vegetables | | ○ | ○ | ○ | ○ | ○ | ○ | ○ |
| Fruits | | ○ | ○ | ○ | ○ | ○ | ○ | ○ |
| Carbohydrates | | ○ | ○ | ○ | ○ | ○ | ○ | ○ |
| Protein/Dairy | | ○ | ○ | ○ | ○ | ○ | ○ | ○ |
| Fats | | ○ | ○ | ○ | ○ | ○ | ○ | ○ |
| Sweets | | ○ | ○ | ○ | ○ | ○ | ○ | ○ |

**DIRECTIONS:**
1. Write your daily serving goals for each food group in the table above.
2. Compare the serving totals that you recorded for each day of the past week with your goals.
3. Check off the circles in the table above if your serving totals have met your goals.

**NEW FOOD I WOULD LIKE TO TRY:**

**NEW WAYS TO ADD ACTIVITY TO MY DAY:**

**REMINDER:** 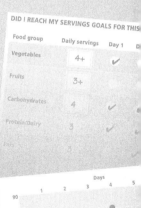 Calculate your weight change in this Review and record it in the Weight Record.

**HOW MANY STEPS A DAY DID I TAKE (IF I USED A PEDOMETER)?**

| Day 1 | Day 2 | Day 3 | Day 4 | Day 5 | Day 6 | Day 7 |
|-------|-------|-------|-------|-------|-------|-------|
|       |       |       |       |       |       |       |

**HOW MANY MINUTES A DAY WAS I ACTIVE?**

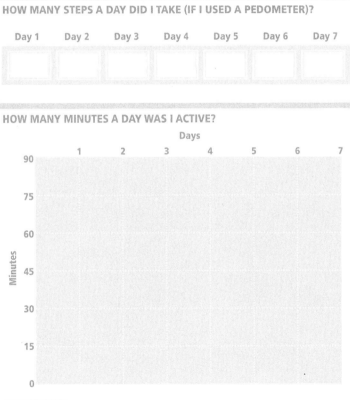

**DIRECTIONS:**
1. Add a dot for your total minutes of activity for each day of last week.
2. Connect each dot on the chart with a line.

See a sample chart to the right. →

DID I REACH MY SERVINGS GOALS FOR THIS

| Food group | Daily servings | Day 1 | D |
|------------|----------------|-------|---|
| Vegetables | 4+ | ✓ | |
| Fruits | 3+ | | |
| Carbohydrates | 4 | ✓ | |
| Protein/Dairy | 3 | ✓ | |
| Fats | 3 | | |

The samples above show how you can fill out your servings goals table and your activity chart for your weekly Review.

| Day | Breakfast | Lunch | Dinner | Snack |
|-----|-----------|-------|--------|-------|
| EXAMPLE | cereal banana | spaghetti fruit salad | tuna wrap baby carrots | crackers and cheese |
| 1 | | | | |
| 2 | | | | |
| 3 | | | | |
| 4 | | | | |
| 5 | | | | |
| 6 | | | | |
| 7 | | | | |

| Exercise and activities | Events and special plans |
|---|---|
| swim class @ 11am<br>walk to work | kids ballgame @ 6pm<br>note: supper will be on the go |
| | |
| | |
| | |
| | |
| | |
| | |
| | |

# WEEK AT A GLANCE

**USING THE PLANNER:**

Organize your plans for meals, activities and exercise in the coming week. Note upcoming events that may affect your weight program, such as travel, eating out, social occasions and vacations.

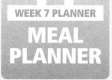

| MAIN MEAL OR MEALS OF THE DAY | HOW MUCH |
|---|---|
| | |

**EASY AS 1, 2, 3:**

This page allows you to check how well a meal meets your recommended servings goals.

1. Write down what you're planning to eat for this meal (or for the entire day).
2. Calculate the number of servings based on how much you're planning to eat.
3. Be sure to include the food items from your menu in your Shopping List.

**PYRAMID SERVINGS FOR THIS MEAL**

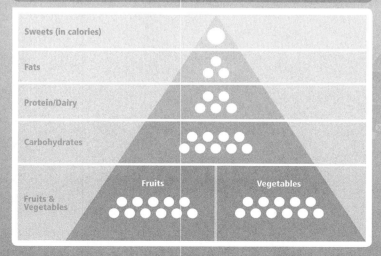

Sweets (in calories)

Fats

Protein/Dairy

Carbohydrates

Fruits

Vegetables

Fruits & Vegetables

◀ Check off the number of servings on the pyramid at left.

WEEK 7 PLANNER

## MEAL PLANNER

| MAIN MEAL OR MEALS OF THE DAY | HOW MUCH |
|---|---|
|  |  |

EASY AS 1, 2, 3:

This page allows you to check how well a meal meets your recommended servings goals.

1. Write down what you're planning to eat for this meal (or for the entire day).
2. Calculate the number of servings based on how much you're planning to eat.
3. Be sure to include the food items from your menu in your Shopping List.

## PYRAMID SERVINGS FOR THIS MEAL

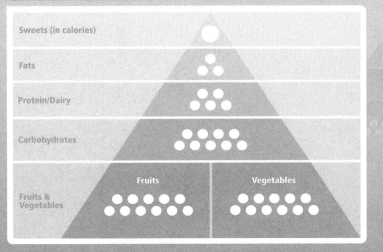

Sweets (in calories)

Fats

Protein/Dairy

Carbohydrates

Fruits & Vegetables

Fruits

Vegetables

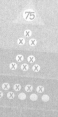

◄ Check off the number of servings on the pyramid at left.

## MENU FOR THE DAY

### BREAKFAST
1 slice whole-grain toast
1½ tbsp. jam
*1 large grapefruit
Calorie-free beverage

| V | F | C | PD | Pt | S |
|---|---|---|----|----|---|
| 0 | 2 | 1 | 0  | 0  | 1 |

### LUNCH
California Burger
*1 small apple
Calorie-free beverage

| V | F | C | PD | Pt | S |
|---|---|---|----|----|---|
| 1 | 1 | 2 | 2  | 1  | 0 |

### DINNER
1 serving Greek Salad
6 whole-grain crackers
Calorie-free beverage

| V | F | C | PD | Pt | S |
|---|---|---|----|----|---|
| 2 | 0 | 1 | 1  | 1  | 0 |

### SNACK
*1 serving favorite vegetable
3 tbsp. fat-free sour cream

| V | F | C | PD | Pt | S |
|---|---|---|----|----|---|
| 1 | 0 | 0 | 0  | 1  | 0 |

*The serving size stated is the minimum amount. Eat as much as you wish.

QUICK TIP:

The menu on this page demonstrates how you can plan your own daily menus. Feel free to include this sample on one of your days.

## LUNCH RECIPE

### California Burger

- Top a 3-ounce, cooked, extra-lean ground beef patty with ½ grilled onion slice, tomato slice and lettuce. Serve on a small whole-grain bun spread with 1 tablespoon reduced-calorie mayonnaise.

## DINNER RECIPE

### Greek Salad

2 C. red and green leaf lettuce
¼ C. diced cucumber
¼ C. diced sweet bell pepper
¼ C. diced carrots
¼ C. crumbled feta cheese
1 slice red onion
2 pitted Kalamata olives
2 pepperoncini peppers
1 tbsp. balsamic vinegar

- Put lettuce in a bowl and toss with diced cucumber, bell pepper and carrots.
- Top salad with feta cheese and onion slice, separated into rings.
- Garnish with Kalamata olives and pepperoncini peppers.
- Drizzle with balsamic vinegar and serve immediately.

| Fresh produce | Whole grains | Meat & dairy |
|---|---|---|
| | | |
| | | |

| Frozen goods | Canned goods | Miscellaneous |
|---|---|---|
| | | |
| | | |

WEEK 7 PLANNER

# SHOPPING LIST

QUICK TIP:

Create your shopping list for the week before going to the grocery store. You'll have all the ingredients on hand at the time you prepare a meal.

| Fresh produce | Whole grains |
|---|---|
| 10 large tomatoes | 8 oz package spaghetti |
| 2 red peppers | 1 loaf rye brea |
| summer squash | 1 package en muffins |
| zucchini | |
| 1 bag baby carrots | bag of pita |
| cherries | |
| 3 grapefruit | |

Add to your Shopping List as you plan your menus for the week.

**TODAY'S DATE:**

**TODAY'S GOAL:**

**NOTES ABOUT TODAY:**

**WHAT I ATE TODAY:**                                    Number of servings per food group

| ⏱ Time | Food item | Amount | V | F | C | PD | Ft | S |
|---------|-----------|--------|---|---|---|----|----|----|
|  |  |  |  |  |  |  |  |  |
|  |  |  |  |  |  |  |  |  |
|  |  |  |  |  |  |  |  |  |
|  |  |  |  |  |  |  |  |  |
|  |  |  |  |  |  |  |  |  |
|  |  |  |  |  |  |  |  |  |
|  |  |  |  |  |  |  |  |  |
|  |  |  |  |  |  |  |  |  |
|  |  |  |  |  |  |  |  |  |
|  |  |  |  |  |  |  |  |  |
|  |  |  |  |  |  |  |  |  |
|  |  |  |  |  |  |  |  |  |
|  |  |  |  |  |  |  |  |  |

**TODAY'S ACTIVITIES:**　🕐 Time

|  |  |
|---|---|
|  |  |
|  |  |
|  |  |
|  |  |
| **Total time (in minutes)** |  |

**MOTIVATION TIP:**
To reduce stress, try organizing your day to avoid conflict and last-minute panic. Tackle unpleasant tasks early and get them over with sooner.

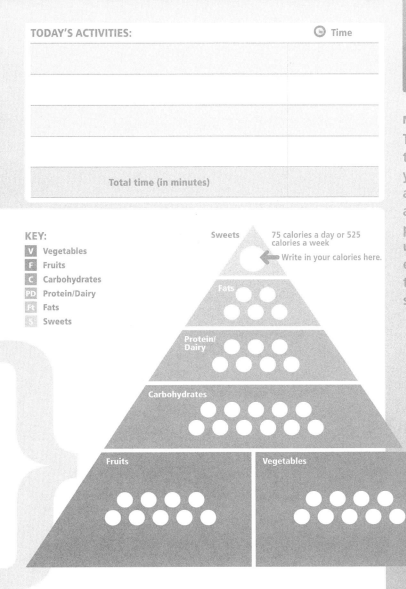

**KEY:**
- V Vegetables
- F Fruits
- C Carbohydrates
- PD Protein/Dairy
- Ft Fats
- S Sweets

Sweets — 75 calories a day or 525 calories a week
← Write in your calories here.

Fats

Protein/Dairy

Carbohydrates

Fruits

Vegetables

**WHAT I ATE TODAY FROM THE PYRAMID:**
Check off the circles in the food group servings above as you record food and beverage items in the table at left. For sweets, give your best estimate of the total number of calories for the day.

**TODAY'S DATE:**

**TODAY'S GOAL:**

**NOTES ABOUT TODAY:**

**WHAT I ATE TODAY:**

Number of servings per food group

| 🕐 Time | Food item | Amount | V | F | C | PD | FT | S |
|--------|-----------|--------|---|---|---|----|----|---|
| | | | | | | | | |
| | | | | | | | | |
| | | | | | | | | |
| | | | | | | | | |
| | | | | | | | | |
| | | | | | | | | |
| | | | | | | | | |
| | | | | | | | | |
| | | | | | | | | |
| | | | | | | | | |
| | | | | | | | | |
| | | | | | | | | |
| | | | | | | | | |

**TODAY'S ACTIVITIES:**

🕐 Time

Total time (in minutes)

**MOTIVATION TIP:**

To cut down on snacking at the movie theater, eat something healthy before you leave home. Drink water or a calorie-free beverage while you're there.

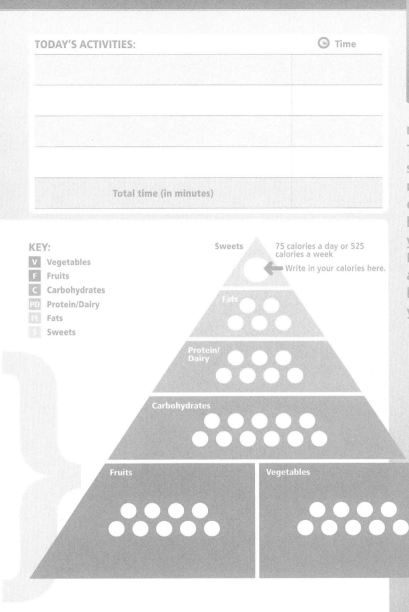

**KEY:**
- V Vegetables
- F Fruits
- C Carbohydrates
- PD Protein/Dairy
- Ft Fats
- S Sweets

Sweets — 75 calories a day or 525 calories a week

← Write in your calories here.

Fats

Protein/Dairy

Carbohydrates

Fruits

Vegetables

**WHAT I ATE TODAY FROM THE PYRAMID:**
Check off the circles in the food group servings above as you record food and beverage items in the table at left. For sweets, give your best estimate of the total number of calories for the day.

**TODAY'S DATE:**

**TODAY'S GOAL:**

**NOTES ABOUT TODAY:**

**WHAT I ATE TODAY:**                     Number of servings per food group

| ⏱ Time | Food item | Amount | V | F | C | PD | Ft | S |
|--------|-----------|--------|---|---|---|----|----|---|
|  |  |  |  |  |  |  |  |  |
|  |  |  |  |  |  |  |  |  |
|  |  |  |  |  |  |  |  |  |
|  |  |  |  |  |  |  |  |  |
|  |  |  |  |  |  |  |  |  |
|  |  |  |  |  |  |  |  |  |
|  |  |  |  |  |  |  |  |  |
|  |  |  |  |  |  |  |  |  |
|  |  |  |  |  |  |  |  |  |
|  |  |  |  |  |  |  |  |  |
|  |  |  |  |  |  |  |  |  |
|  |  |  |  |  |  |  |  |  |

## TODAY'S ACTIVITIES:

🕐 Time

|  |  |
|---|---|
|  |  |
|  |  |
|  |  |
|  |  |
| **Total time (in minutes)** |  |

**MOTIVATION TIP:**

Mix things up when you exercise. Don't feel tied to just one type of activity, such as walking. Occasionally, try biking or swimming instead.

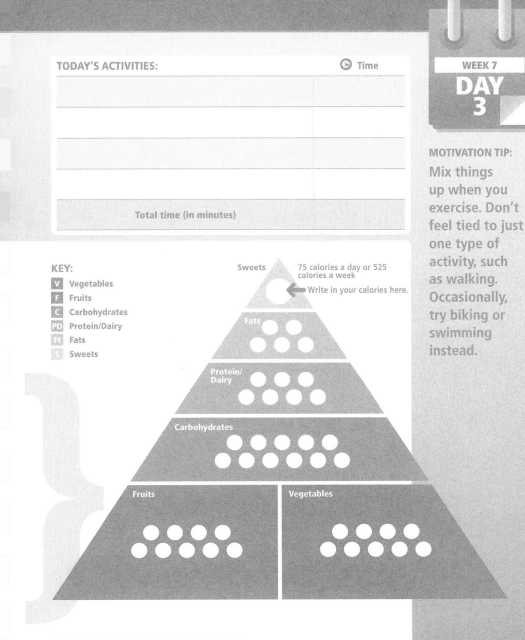

**KEY:**

- **V** Vegetables
- **F** Fruits
- **C** Carbohydrates
- **PD** Protein/Dairy
- **Ft** Fats
- **S** Sweets

Sweets — 75 calories a day or 525 calories a week

Write in your calories here.

Fats

Protein/Dairy

Carbohydrates

Fruits

Vegetables

## WHAT I ATE TODAY FROM THE PYRAMID:

Check off the circles in the food group servings above as you record food and beverage items in the table at left. For sweets, give your best estimate of the total number of calories for the day.

**TODAY'S DATE:**

**TODAY'S GOAL:**

**NOTES ABOUT TODAY:**

**WHAT I ATE TODAY:**                                    Number of servings per food group

| ⏱ Time | Food item | Amount | V | F | C | PD | Ft | S |
|---------|-----------|--------|---|---|---|----|----|---|
|         |           |        |   |   |   |    |    |   |
|         |           |        |   |   |   |    |    |   |
|         |           |        |   |   |   |    |    |   |
|         |           |        |   |   |   |    |    |   |
|         |           |        |   |   |   |    |    |   |
|         |           |        |   |   |   |    |    |   |
|         |           |        |   |   |   |    |    |   |
|         |           |        |   |   |   |    |    |   |
|         |           |        |   |   |   |    |    |   |
|         |           |        |   |   |   |    |    |   |
|         |           |        |   |   |   |    |    |   |
|         |           |        |   |   |   |    |    |   |

**TODAY'S ACTIVITIES:**

🕐 **Time**

|  |  |
|---|---|
|  |  |
|  |  |
|  |  |
|  |  |
| Total time (in minutes) |  |

**MOTIVATION TIP:**
Consider growing some of your own produce. It's not as hard as you may think. If you don't have space for a garden plot, you can grow items such as tomatoes and peppers in outdoor pots.

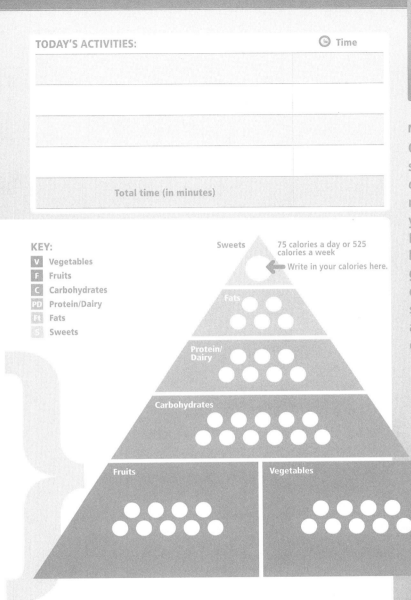

**KEY:**
- V  Vegetables
- F  Fruits
- C  Carbohydrates
- PD Protein/Dairy
- Ft Fats
- S  Sweets

Sweets — 75 calories a day or 525 calories a week

← Write in your calories here.

Fats

Protein/Dairy

Carbohydrates

Fruits

Vegetables

**WHAT I ATE TODAY FROM THE PYRAMID:**
Check off the circles in the food group servings above as you record food and beverage items in the table at left. For sweets, give your best estimate of the total number of calories for the day.

**TODAY'S DATE:**

**TODAY'S GOAL:**

**NOTES ABOUT TODAY:**

**WHAT I ATE TODAY:**      Number of servings per food group

| Time | Food item | Amount | V | F | C | PD | Ft | S |
|------|-----------|--------|---|---|---|----|----|----|
|  |  |  |  |  |  |  |  |  |
|  |  |  |  |  |  |  |  |  |
|  |  |  |  |  |  |  |  |  |
|  |  |  |  |  |  |  |  |  |
|  |  |  |  |  |  |  |  |  |
|  |  |  |  |  |  |  |  |  |
|  |  |  |  |  |  |  |  |  |
|  |  |  |  |  |  |  |  |  |
|  |  |  |  |  |  |  |  |  |
|  |  |  |  |  |  |  |  |  |

## TODAY'S ACTIVITIES:

🕐 Time

| | |
|---|---|
| | |
| | |
| | |
| Total time (in minutes) | |

**MOTIVATION TIP:**

Counteract all-or-nothing thinking. Try not to label a food as being either "good" or "bad." You can eat most foods in moderation. It's even OK to have dessert once in a while.

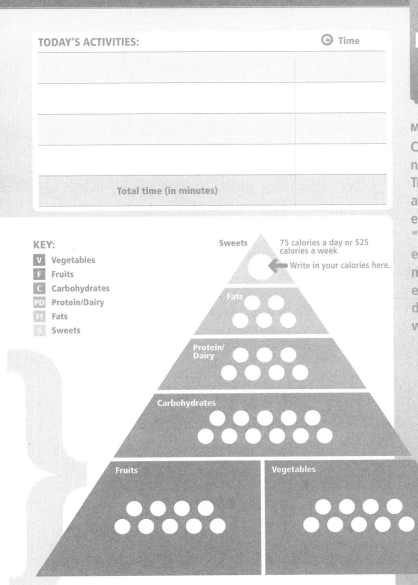

**KEY:**

- **V** Vegetables
- **F** Fruits
- **C** Carbohydrates
- **PD** Protein/Dairy
- **Ft** Fats
- **S** Sweets

Sweets — 75 calories a day or 525 calories a week

Write in your calories here.

Fats

Protein/Dairy

Carbohydrates

Fruits

Vegetables

## WHAT I ATE TODAY FROM THE PYRAMID:

Check off the circles in the food group servings above as you record food and beverage items in the table at left. For sweets, give your best estimate of the total number of calories for the day.

**TODAY'S DATE:**

**TODAY'S GOAL:**

**NOTES ABOUT TODAY:**

**WHAT I ATE TODAY:**

Number of servings per food group

| Time | Food item | Amount | V | F | C | PD | Ft | S |
|------|-----------|--------|---|---|---|----|----|---|
|      |           |        |   |   |   |    |    |   |
|      |           |        |   |   |   |    |    |   |
|      |           |        |   |   |   |    |    |   |
|      |           |        |   |   |   |    |    |   |
|      |           |        |   |   |   |    |    |   |
|      |           |        |   |   |   |    |    |   |
|      |           |        |   |   |   |    |    |   |
|      |           |        |   |   |   |    |    |   |
|      |           |        |   |   |   |    |    |   |
|      |           |        |   |   |   |    |    |   |
|      |           |        |   |   |   |    |    |   |

**TODAY'S ACTIVITIES:**                              🕐 Time

| | |
|---|---|
| | |
| | |
| | |
| **Total time (in minutes)** | |

**MOTIVATION TIP:**
Try to build your self-esteem. Don't hide behind oversized, drab clothing. Dress in clothing that makes you feel good about yourself.

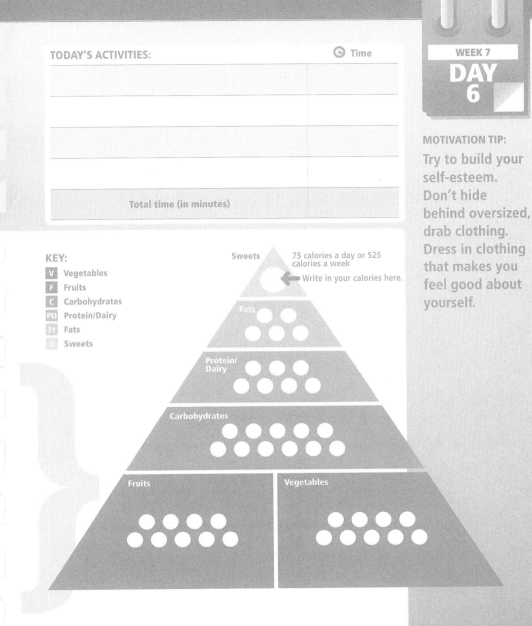

**KEY:**
- **V** Vegetables
- **F** Fruits
- **C** Carbohydrates
- **PD** Protein/Dairy
- **Ft** Fats
- **S** Sweets

Sweets — 75 calories a day or 525 calories a week
← Write in your calories here.

Fats

Protein/Dairy

Carbohydrates

Fruits

Vegetables

**WHAT I ATE TODAY FROM THE PYRAMID:**
Check off the circles in the food group servings above as you record food and beverage items in the table at left. For sweets, give your best estimate of the total number of calories for the day.

**TODAY'S DATE:**

**TODAY'S GOAL:**

**NOTES ABOUT TODAY:**
It's weigh-in day ~ record my weight in the weekly Review and the Weight Record.

**WHAT I ATE TODAY:**

Number of servings per food group

| Time | Food item | Amount | V | F | C | PD | Ft | S |
|------|-----------|--------|---|---|---|----|----|---|
|      |           |        |   |   |   |    |    |   |
|      |           |        |   |   |   |    |    |   |
|      |           |        |   |   |   |    |    |   |
|      |           |        |   |   |   |    |    |   |
|      |           |        |   |   |   |    |    |   |
|      |           |        |   |   |   |    |    |   |
|      |           |        |   |   |   |    |    |   |
|      |           |        |   |   |   |    |    |   |
|      |           |        |   |   |   |    |    |   |
|      |           |        |   |   |   |    |    |   |

**TODAY'S ACTIVITIES:**

🕐 Time

Total time (in minutes)

**REMINDER:**

Record your weight for today in the weekly Review and the Weight Record.

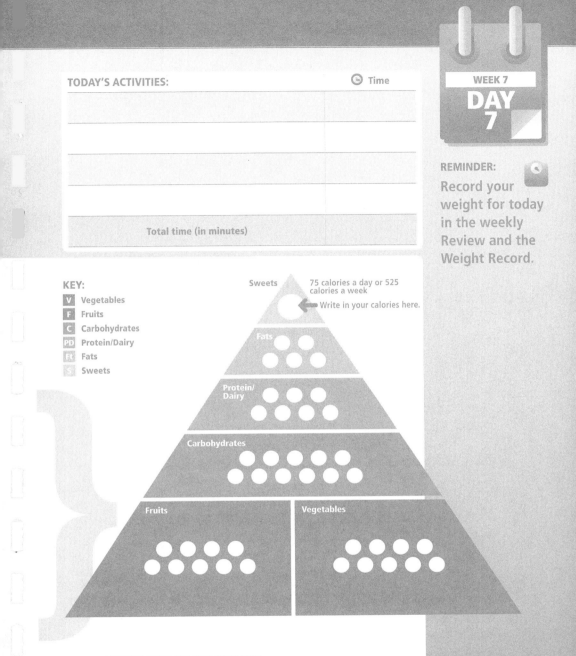

**KEY:**

| V | Vegetables |
| F | Fruits |
| C | Carbohydrates |
| PD | Protein/Dairy |
| R | Fats |
| S | Sweets |

Sweets — 75 calories a day or 525 calories a week
◀ Write in your calories here.

Fats

Protein/Dairy

Carbohydrates

Fruits

Vegetables

**WHAT I ATE TODAY FROM THE PYRAMID:**

Check off the circles in the food group servings above as you record food and beverage items in the table at left. For sweets, give your best estimate of the total number of calories for the day.

My start weight ☐
Minus my weight today ☐
= Equals my weight change ☐

**I FEEL:**
- ○ Terrific
- ○ Good
- ○ So-so
- ○ Discouraged
- ○ Like giving up

**I'M MOST PROUD OF:**

**WHAT WORKED WELL:**

**WHAT DIDN'T WORK AS WELL:**

**DID I REACH MY SERVINGS GOALS FOR THIS WEEK?**

| Food group | Daily servings | Day 1 | Day 2 | Day 3 | Day 4 | Day 5 | Day 6 | Day 7 |
|---|---|---|---|---|---|---|---|---|
| Vegetables | ☐ | ○ | ○ | ○ | ○ | ○ | ○ | ○ |
| Fruits | ☐ | ○ | ○ | ○ | ○ | ○ | ○ | ○ |
| Carbohydrates | ☐ | ○ | ○ | ○ | ○ | ○ | ○ | ○ |
| Protein/Dairy | ☐ | ○ | ○ | ○ | ○ | ○ | ○ | ○ |
| Fats | ☐ | ○ | ○ | ○ | ○ | ○ | ○ | ○ |
| Sweets | ☐ | ○ | ○ | ○ | ○ | ○ | ○ | ○ |

**DIRECTIONS:**
1. Write your daily serving goals for each food group in the table above.
2. Compare the serving totals that you recorded for each day of the past week with your goals.
3. Check off the circles in the table above if your serving totals have met your goals.

**NEW FOOD I WOULD LIKE TO TRY:**

**NEW WAYS TO ADD ACTIVITY TO MY DAY:**

**REMINDER:** Calculate your weight change in this Review and record it in the Weight Record.

**HOW MANY STEPS A DAY DID I TAKE (IF I USED A PEDOMETER)?**

| Day 1 | Day 2 | Day 3 | Day 4 | Day 5 | Day 6 | Day 7 |
|-------|-------|-------|-------|-------|-------|-------|
|       |       |       |       |       |       |       |

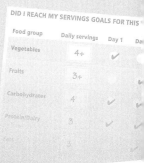

**DID I REACH MY SERVINGS GOALS FOR THIS**

| Food group | Daily servings | Day 1 | Da |
|------------|----------------|-------|-----|
| Vegetables | 4+ | ✓ |  |
| Fruits | 3+ |  |  |
| Carbohydrates | 4 | ✓ |  |
| Protein/Dairy | 3 | ✓ |  |
| Fats | 3 |  | ✓ |

**HOW MANY MINUTES A DAY WAS I ACTIVE?**

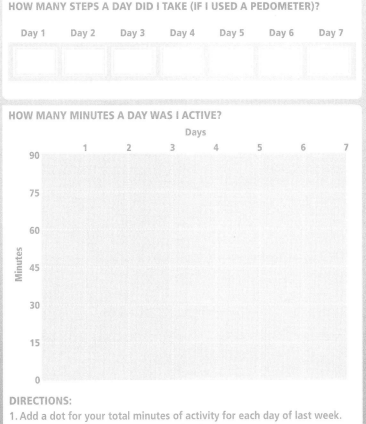

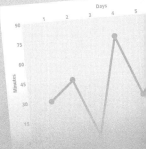

**DIRECTIONS:**
1. Add a dot for your total minutes of activity for each day of last week.
2. Connect each dot on the chart with a line.

See a sample chart to the right. ➜

The samples above show how you can fill out your servings goals table and your activity chart for your weekly Review.

# Live It!

**WEEK 8 PLANNER** ▸ **WEEK AT A GLANCE**

| Day | Breakfast | Lunch | Dinner | Snack |
|---|---|---|---|---|
| EXAMPLE | cereal banana | spaghetti fruit salad | tuna wrap baby carrots | crackers and cheese |
| 1 | | | | |
| 2 | | | | |
| 3 | | | | |
| 4 | | | | |
| 5 | | | | |
| 6 | | | | |
| 7 | | | | |

| Exercise and activities | Events and special plans |
|---|---|
| swim class @ 11am<br>walk to work | kids ballgame @ 6pm<br>note: supper will be on the go |
|  |  |
|  |  |
|  |  |
|  |  |
|  |  |
|  |  |
|  |  |

**USING THE PLANNER:**

Organize your plans for meals, activities and exercise in the coming week. Note upcoming events that may affect your weight program, such as travel, eating out, social occasions and vacations.

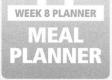

| MAIN MEAL OR MEALS OF THE DAY | HOW MUCH |
|---|---|
| | |

**EASY AS 1, 2, 3:**

This page allows you to check how well a meal meets your recommended servings goals.

1. Write down what you're planning to eat for this meal (or for the entire day).

2. Calculate the number of servings based on how much you're planning to eat.

3. Be sure to include the food items from your menu in your Shopping List.

## PYRAMID SERVINGS FOR THIS MEAL

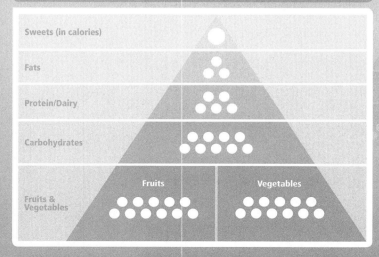

| | |
|---|---|
| Sweets (in calories) | |
| Fats | |
| Protein/Dairy | |
| Carbohydrates | |
| Fruits & Vegetables | Fruits / Vegetables |

◄ Check off the number of servings on the pyramid at left.

WEEK 8 PLANNER

# MEAL PLANNER

| MAIN MEAL OR MEALS OF THE DAY | HOW MUCH |
|---|---|
|  |  |

**EASY AS 1, 2, 3:**

This page allows you to check how well a meal meets your recommended servings goals.

1. Write down what you're planning to eat for this meal (or for the entire day).

2. Calculate the number of servings based on how much you're planning to eat.

3. Be sure to include the food items from your menu in your Shopping List.

## PYRAMID SERVINGS FOR THIS MEAL

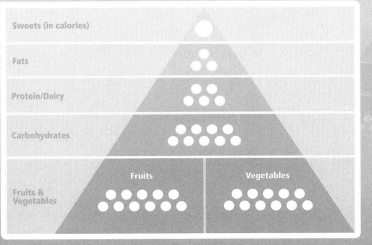

Sweets (in calories)

Fats

Protein/Dairy

Carbohydrates

Fruits & Vegetables — Fruits — Vegetables

◀ Check off the number of servings on the pyramid at left.

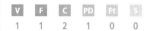
## MENU FOR THE DAY

### BREAKFAST
Breakfast Burrito
*1 medium orange
Calorie-free beverage

| V | F | C | PD | Ft | S |
|---|---|---|----|----|---|
| 1 | 1 | 2 | 1  | 0  | 0 |

### LUNCH
Spinach Fruit Salad
2 tbsp. low-calorie French dressing
1 c. skim milk
8 whole peanuts or 4 whole cashews
Calorie-free beverage

| V | F | C | PD | Ft | S |
|---|---|---|----|----|---|
| 2 | 1 | 0 | 1  | 2  | 0 |

### DINNER
3 oz. fish or shrimp, broiled or grilled
⅔ c. cooked brown rice
*1 c. steamed broccoli
*2 c. lettuce
2 tbsp. reduced-calorie salad dressing
*1 c. mixed berries
Calorie-free beverage

| V | F | C | PD | Ft | S |
|---|---|---|----|----|---|
| 2 | 1 | 2 | 1  | 1  | 0 |

### SNACK
*1 serving favorite fruit

| V | F | C | PD | Ft | S |
|---|---|---|----|----|---|
| 0 | 1 | 0 | 0  | 0  | 0 |

*The serving size stated is the minimum amount. Eat as much as you wish.

QUICK TIP:
The menu on this page demonstrates how you can plan your own daily menus. Feel free to include this sample on one of your days.

## BREAKFAST RECIPE

### Breakfast Burrito

- Sauté ½ cup chopped tomato, 2 tablespoons chopped onion and ¼ cup canned corn with some of its liquid. Add ¼ cup egg substitute and scramble with vegetables. Spread on a fat-free tortilla, roll up the tortilla, and top with 2 tablespoons of salsa.

## LUNCH RECIPE

### Spinach Fruit Salad

- Top 2 cups of baby spinach with ½ cup green pepper strips and water chestnuts, and ½ cup mandarin orange sections.

WEEK 8 PLANNER

# SHOPPING LIST

| Fresh produce | Whole grains | Meat & dairy |
| --- | --- | --- |
| | | |

| Frozen goods | Canned goods | Miscellaneous |
| --- | --- | --- |
| | | |

QUICK TIP:

Create your shopping list for the week before going to the grocery store. You'll have all the ingredients on hand at the time you prepare a meal.

| Fresh produce | Whole grains |
| --- | --- |
| 10 large tomatoes | 8 oz package spaghetti |
| 2 red peppers | 1 loaf rye bread |
| summer squash | 1 package en muffins |
| zucchini | |
| 1 bag baby carrots | bag of pita |
| cherries | |
| 5 grapefruit | |

Add to your Shopping List as you plan your menus for the week.

**TODAY'S DATE:**

**TODAY'S GOAL:**

**NOTES ABOUT TODAY:**

**WHAT I ATE TODAY:**                                    Number of servings per food group

| ⏱ Time | Food item | Amount | V | F | C | PD | Ft | S |
|---------|-----------|--------|---|---|---|----|----|----|
|  |  |  |  |  |  |  |  |  |
|  |  |  |  |  |  |  |  |  |
|  |  |  |  |  |  |  |  |  |
|  |  |  |  |  |  |  |  |  |
|  |  |  |  |  |  |  |  |  |
|  |  |  |  |  |  |  |  |  |
|  |  |  |  |  |  |  |  |  |
|  |  |  |  |  |  |  |  |  |
|  |  |  |  |  |  |  |  |  |
|  |  |  |  |  |  |  |  |  |
|  |  |  |  |  |  |  |  |  |

**TODAY'S ACTIVITIES:**                                    🕐 Time

|  |  |
|--|--|
|  |  |
|  |  |
|  |  |
|  |  |
| **Total time (in minutes)** |  |

**MOTIVATION TIP:**

If you can stay focused on a healthy lifestyle, the weight will take care of itself. That includes a balanced diet, daily physical activity, getting enough sleep and managing stress.

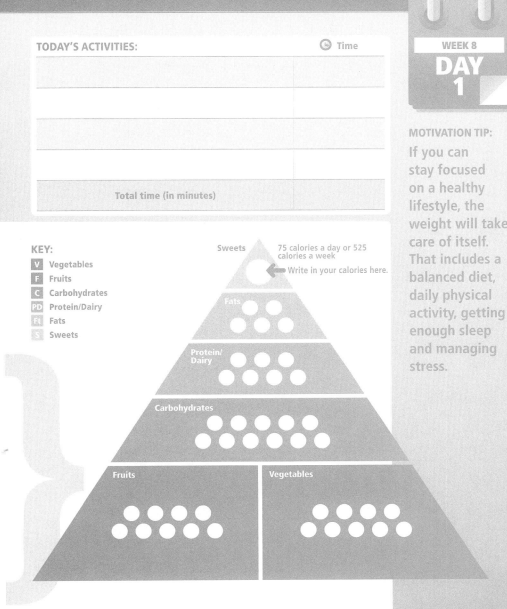

**KEY:**

- **V** Vegetables
- **F** Fruits
- **C** Carbohydrates
- **PD** Protein/Dairy
- **Ft** Fats
- **S** Sweets

Sweets — 75 calories a day or 525 calories a week

⬅ Write in your calories here.

Fats

Protein/Dairy

Carbohydrates

Fruits

Vegetables

**WHAT I ATE TODAY FROM THE PYRAMID:**

Check off the circles in the food group servings above as you record food and beverage items in the table at left. For sweets, give your best estimate of the total number of calories for the day.

**TODAY'S DATE:**

**TODAY'S GOAL:**

**NOTES ABOUT TODAY:**

**WHAT I ATE TODAY:**

Number of servings per food group

| 🕐 Time | Food item | Amount | V | F | C | PD | Ft | S |
|---------|-----------|--------|---|---|---|----|----|---|
|         |           |        |   |   |   |    |    |   |
|         |           |        |   |   |   |    |    |   |
|         |           |        |   |   |   |    |    |   |
|         |           |        |   |   |   |    |    |   |
|         |           |        |   |   |   |    |    |   |
|         |           |        |   |   |   |    |    |   |
|         |           |        |   |   |   |    |    |   |
|         |           |        |   |   |   |    |    |   |
|         |           |        |   |   |   |    |    |   |
|         |           |        |   |   |   |    |    |   |
|         |           |        |   |   |   |    |    |   |

**TODAY'S ACTIVITIES:**

🕐 Time

| | |
|---|---|
| Total time (in minutes) | |

**MOTIVATION TIP:**

To continue losing weight or maintaining the weight you have, keep doing whatever worked for you in the past. You can always adapt tried-and-true strategies to meet changing circumstances.

**KEY:**

- **V** Vegetables
- **F** Fruits
- **C** Carbohydrates
- **PD** Protein/Dairy
- **Ft** Fats
- **S** Sweets

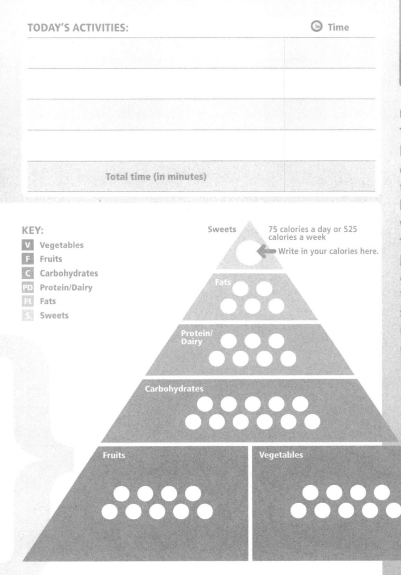

Sweets — 75 calories a day or 525 calories a week

Write in your calories here.

Fats

Protein/Dairy

Carbohydrates

Fruits

Vegetables

**WHAT I ATE TODAY FROM THE PYRAMID:**

Check off the circles in the food group servings above as you record food and beverage items in the table at left. For sweets, give your best estimate of the total number of calories for the day.

**TODAY'S DATE:**

**TODAY'S GOAL:**

**NOTES ABOUT TODAY:**

**WHAT I ATE TODAY:**

Number of servings per food group

| Time | Food item | Amount | V | F | C | PD | Ft | S |
|------|-----------|--------|---|---|---|----|----|----|
| | | | | | | | | |
| | | | | | | | | |
| | | | | | | | | |
| | | | | | | | | |
| | | | | | | | | |
| | | | | | | | | |
| | | | | | | | | |
| | | | | | | | | |
| | | | | | | | | |
| | | | | | | | | |
| | | | | | | | | |
| | | | | | | | | |
| | | | | | | | | |

**TODAY'S ACTIVITIES:**  🕐 Time

|  |  |
|---|---|
|  |  |
|  |  |
|  |  |
|  |  |
| **Total time (in minutes)** |  |

**MOTIVATION TIP:**
What you do to maintain your weight should be things you look forward to doing. You want to make weight control enjoyable and comforting, not unpleasant and tiresome.

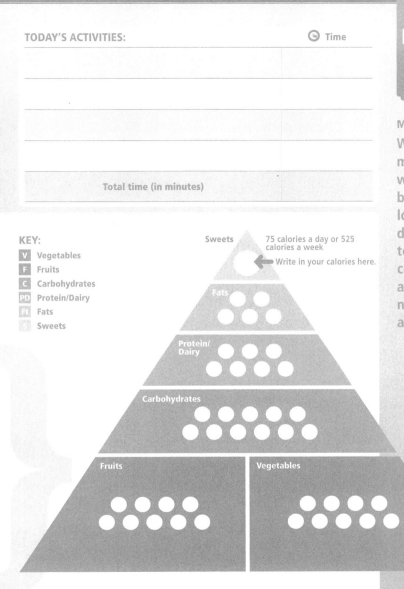

**KEY:**
- **V** Vegetables
- **F** Fruits
- **C** Carbohydrates
- **PD** Protein/Dairy
- **Ft** Fats
- **S** Sweets

Sweets — 75 calories a day or 525 calories a week
← Write in your calories here.

Fats

Protein/Dairy

Carbohydrates

Fruits

Vegetables

**WHAT I ATE TODAY FROM THE PYRAMID:**
Check off the circles in the food group servings above as you record food and beverage items in the table at left. For sweets, give your best estimate of the total number of calories for the day.

**TODAY'S DATE:**

**TODAY'S GOAL:**

**NOTES ABOUT TODAY:**

**WHAT I ATE TODAY:**

Number of servings per food group

| Time | Food item | Amount | V | F | C | PD | Pt | S |
|------|-----------|--------|---|---|---|----|----|---|
|  |  |  |  |  |  |  |  |  |
|  |  |  |  |  |  |  |  |  |
|  |  |  |  |  |  |  |  |  |
|  |  |  |  |  |  |  |  |  |
|  |  |  |  |  |  |  |  |  |
|  |  |  |  |  |  |  |  |  |
|  |  |  |  |  |  |  |  |  |
|  |  |  |  |  |  |  |  |  |
|  |  |  |  |  |  |  |  |  |
|  |  |  |  |  |  |  |  |  |
|  |  |  |  |  |  |  |  |  |
|  |  |  |  |  |  |  |  |  |

**TODAY'S ACTIVITIES:**

🕐 Time

| | |
|---|---|
| | |
| | |
| | |
| | |
| Total time (in minutes) | |

**MOTIVATION TIP:**

Regardless of how much weight you've lost, the fact that you've stayed with the program and continued to use the journal for this long is an important achievement.

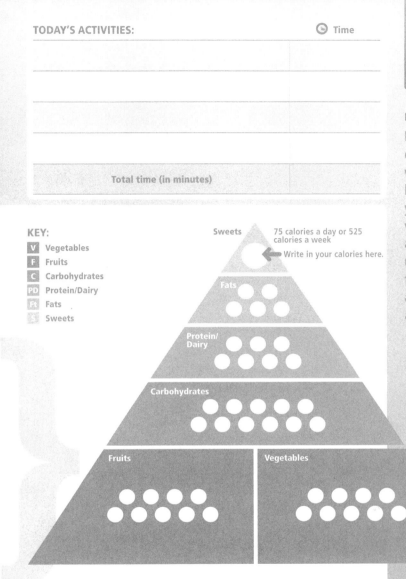

**KEY:**
- V Vegetables
- F Fruits
- C Carbohydrates
- PD Protein/Dairy
- Ft Fats
- Sweets

Sweets — 75 calories a day or 525 calories a week
← Write in your calories here.

Fats

Protein/Dairy

Carbohydrates

Fruits   Vegetables

**WHAT I ATE TODAY FROM THE PYRAMID:**

Check off the circles in the food group servings above as you record food and beverage items in the table at left. For sweets, give your best estimate of the total number of calories for the day.

**TODAY'S DATE:**

**TODAY'S GOAL:**

**NOTES ABOUT TODAY:**

**WHAT I ATE TODAY:**　　　　　　　　　　Number of servings per food group

| Time | Food item | Amount | V | F | C | PD | Pt | S |
|------|-----------|--------|---|---|---|----|----|---|
|  |  |  |  |  |  |  |  |  |
|  |  |  |  |  |  |  |  |  |
|  |  |  |  |  |  |  |  |  |
|  |  |  |  |  |  |  |  |  |
|  |  |  |  |  |  |  |  |  |
|  |  |  |  |  |  |  |  |  |
|  |  |  |  |  |  |  |  |  |
|  |  |  |  |  |  |  |  |  |
|  |  |  |  |  |  |  |  |  |
|  |  |  |  |  |  |  |  |  |

**TODAY'S ACTIVITIES:**

🕐 Time

| | |
|---|---|
| | |
| | |
| | |
| | |
| **Total time (in minutes)** | |

**MOTIVATION TIP:**
Make a list of the people you most admire. This may include parents, children, educators, scientists and world leaders. Do they have perfect bodies? Does it really matter?

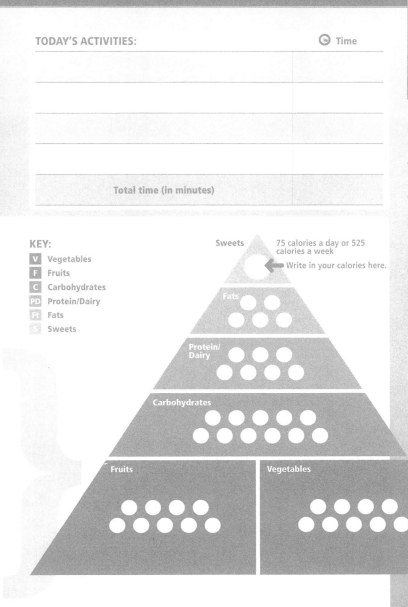

**KEY:**
- **V** Vegetables
- **F** Fruits
- **C** Carbohydrates
- **PD** Protein/Dairy
- **Ft** Fats
- **S** Sweets

Sweets — 75 calories a day or 525 calories a week
— Write in your calories here.

Fats

Protein/Dairy

Carbohydrates

Fruits

Vegetables

**WHAT I ATE TODAY FROM THE PYRAMID:**
Check off the circles in the food group servings above as you record food and beverage items in the table at left. For sweets, give your best estimate of the total number of calories for the day.

**TODAY'S DATE:**

**TODAY'S GOAL:**

**NOTES ABOUT TODAY:**

**WHAT I ATE TODAY:**

Number of servings per food group

| 🕐 Time | Food item | Amount | V | F | C | PD | Ft | S |
|---------|-----------|--------|---|---|---|----|----|---|
| | | | | | | | | |
| | | | | | | | | |
| | | | | | | | | |
| | | | | | | | | |
| | | | | | | | | |
| | | | | | | | | |
| | | | | | | | | |
| | | | | | | | | |
| | | | | | | | | |
| | | | | | | | | |
| | | | | | | | | |
| | | | | | | | | |

**TODAY'S ACTIVITIES:**

🕐 Time

Total time (in minutes)

**MOTIVATION TIP:**
Doing something nice for someone else can boost your self-esteem. Send a card or flowers to someone, offer assistance or do volunteer work in your community.

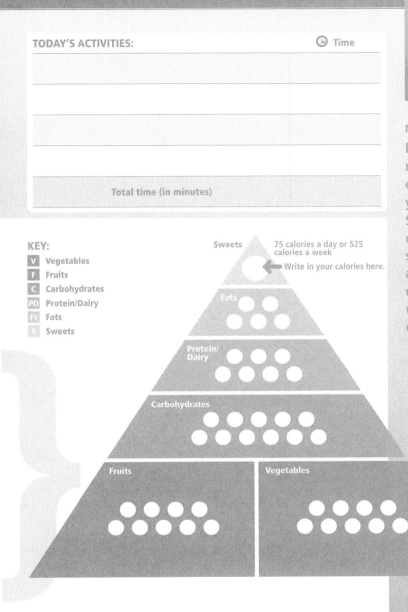

**KEY:**
- **V** Vegetables
- **F** Fruits
- **C** Carbohydrates
- **PD** Protein/Dairy
- **Ft** Fats
- **S** Sweets

Sweets — 75 calories a day or 525 calories a week

Write in your calories here.

Fats

Protein/Dairy

Carbohydrates

Fruits

Vegetables

**WHAT I ATE TODAY FROM THE PYRAMID:**
Check off the circles in the food group servings above as you record food and beverage items in the table at left. For sweets, give your best estimate of the total number of calories for the day.

**TODAY'S DATE:**

**TODAY'S GOAL:**

**NOTES ABOUT TODAY:**
It's weigh-in day ~ record my weight in the weekly Review and the Weight Record.

**WHAT I ATE TODAY:**                                        Number of servings per food group

| Time | Food item | Amount | V | F | C | PD | Ft | S |
|------|-----------|--------|---|---|---|----|----|---|
|  |  |  |  |  |  |  |  |  |
|  |  |  |  |  |  |  |  |  |
|  |  |  |  |  |  |  |  |  |
|  |  |  |  |  |  |  |  |  |
|  |  |  |  |  |  |  |  |  |
|  |  |  |  |  |  |  |  |  |
|  |  |  |  |  |  |  |  |  |
|  |  |  |  |  |  |  |  |  |
|  |  |  |  |  |  |  |  |  |
|  |  |  |  |  |  |  |  |  |
|  |  |  |  |  |  |  |  |  |
|  |  |  |  |  |  |  |  |  |

**TODAY'S ACTIVITIES:**                                🕐 Time

Total time (in minutes)

**REMINDER:**
Record your
weight for today
in the weekly
Review and the
Weight Record.

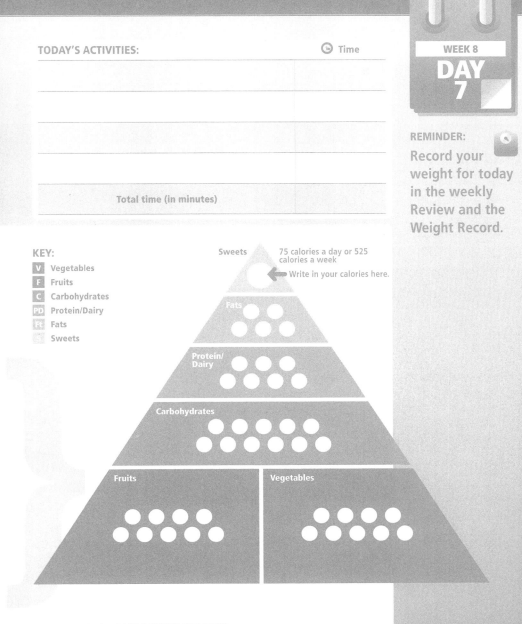

**KEY:**
- **V** Vegetables
- **F** Fruits
- **C** Carbohydrates
- **PD** Protein/Dairy
- **Ft** Fats
- Sweets

Sweets · 75 calories a day or 525 calories a week
← Write in your calories here.

Fats

Protein/Dairy

Carbohydrates

Fruits

Vegetables

**WHAT I ATE TODAY FROM THE PYRAMID:**
Check off the circles in the food group servings above as you record
food and beverage items in the table at left. For sweets, give your best
estimate of the total number of calories for the day.

**My start weight**

**Minus my weight today**

**= Equals my weight change**

**I FEEL:**
- Terrific
- Good
- So-so
- Discouraged
- Like giving up

**I'M MOST PROUD OF:**

**WHAT WORKED WELL:**

**WHAT DIDN'T WORK AS WELL:**

**DID I REACH MY SERVINGS GOALS FOR THIS WEEK?**

| Food group | Daily servings | Day 1 | Day 2 | Day 3 | Day 4 | Day 5 | Day 6 | Day 7 |
|---|---|---|---|---|---|---|---|---|
| Vegetables | | ○ | ○ | ○ | ○ | ○ | ○ | ○ |
| Fruits | | ○ | ○ | ○ | ○ | ○ | ○ | ○ |
| Carbohydrates | | ○ | ○ | ○ | ○ | ○ | ○ | ○ |
| Protein/Dairy | | ○ | ○ | ○ | ○ | ○ | ○ | ○ |
| Fats | | ○ | ○ | ○ | ○ | ○ | ○ | ○ |
| Sweets | | ○ | ○ | ○ | ○ | ○ | ○ | ○ |

**DIRECTIONS:**
1. Write your daily serving goals for each food group in the table above.
2. Compare the serving totals that you recorded for each day of the past week with your goals.
3. Check off the circles in the table above if your serving totals have met your goals.

**NEW FOOD I WOULD LIKE TO TRY:**

**REMINDER:** Calculate your weight change in this Review and record it in the Weight Record.

**NEW WAYS TO ADD ACTIVITY TO MY DAY:**

**HOW MANY STEPS A DAY DID I TAKE (IF I USED A PEDOMETER)?**

| Day 1 | Day 2 | Day 3 | Day 4 | Day 5 | Day 6 | Day 7 |
|-------|-------|-------|-------|-------|-------|-------|
|       |       |       |       |       |       |       |

**HOW MANY MINUTES A DAY WAS I ACTIVE?**

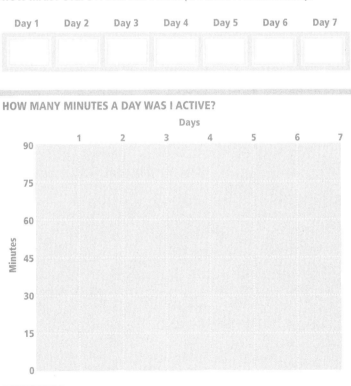

**DID I REACH MY SERVINGS GOALS FOR THIS**

| Food group | Daily servings | Day 1 | |
|------------|---------------|-------|---|
| Vegetables | 4+ | ✓ | |
| Fruits | 3+ | | |
| Carbohydrates | 4 | ✓ | |
| Protein/Dairy | 3 | ✓ | |
| Fats | | | |

**DIRECTIONS:**
1. Add a dot for your total minutes of activity for each day of last week.
2. Connect each dot on the chart with a line.

See a sample chart to the right. →

The samples above show how you can fill out your servings goals table and your activity chart for your weekly Review.

# Making healthy weight a lifetime commitment

Think about the goals you set for yourself at the start of *The Mayo Clinic Diet*. Ten weeks later, do the results meet your expectations?

Judging your progress strictly in terms of the numbers — your weight when you started compared to your weight now — may satisfy you or you end up feeling disappointed. Many people believe they can never lose enough weight, producing an endless cycle of "dieting."

Weight control isn't only about the number of pounds you lose. Here's hoping that *The Mayo Clinic Diet* has given you much more.

Consider that, because of your effort, you're now eating better and you're more active since you started *The Mayo Clinic Diet*. Think about the new strategies you've learned to help overcome obstacles and change unhealthy behaviors. Recall all the foods and recipes you've sampled and enjoyed. All of these changes have combined to make you healthier.

Any amount of weight you've lost, no matter how small, is a step toward a healthier you. At this time, if you feel that you need to lose more weight, you can continue doing what you've been doing. If you're satisfied with the weight you've lost, then your attention turns to keeping those pounds off.

## Strategies for a lifetime

Regardless of which path you choose to take — losing more weight or staying at the weight you have — *The Mayo Clinic Diet* has given you the resources you'll need to achieve your weight goal.

Here are basic guidelines that may help you incorporate what you've learned from *The Mayo Clinic Diet* into a lifetime of healthy living:

### Stick to the basics

Continue to focus on maintaining a healthy lifestyle, and the weight will take care of itself. Stick to a balanced diet, moderate portions and daily physical activity. Get enough sleep and try to manage stress. Remember that these factors are something that everyone should strive to do in life, not just individuals who are intent on losing weight.

### Persistence pays off

Keep doing whatever worked for you in the past. Adapt these strategies to new situations. Vary or add to them to make your program more stimulating or challenging.

Your ultimate goal is to incorporate the new, healthy behaviors that you've learned in the diet into your daily life. You don't want to set them aside after 10 weeks and revert back to your old ways of doing things.

## Make it enjoyable

The things you do to maintain your weight should be things that you look forward to doing. You want them to be enjoyable and comforting, not unpleasant and tiresome. As soon as you start finding excuses or dragging your feet, these new behaviors will be quickly cast aside.

## Keep a long-term perspective

Regardless of how many pounds you may have lost, the fact that you've stayed with the program may be your most important achievement.

It's important to consider weight control beyond a 10-week or 10-month or even 10-year period. It's for a lifetime. And no matter what your expectations may be, by staying committed, you'll reach your goal — perhaps sooner than you think.

## Give yourself credit

Acknowledge the vital role you've played in making your program a success. It was your commitment to losing weight that got you started. It was your energy and persistence that kept you going. You should now have the tools and experience to continue on. Giving yourself credit for what you've accomplished helps raise your confidence level so that you can manage whatever challenges may come along in the future.

## Looking forward

In the months and years ahead, take time occasionally to reconfirm your commitment to weight control. Review your reasons for wanting a healthy weight and the benefits you receive from a healthier lifestyle.

Don't ignore negative feelings or emotions that you may have regarding your efforts — try to determine their causes and look for solutions. Over time, adapt your program or include different strategies in light of changing needs and circumstances.

You've used weigh-ins throughout the 10 weeks of *The Mayo Clinic Diet Journal* to track your progress and keep you motivated. You might find it helpful to continue keeping a weight record, even if you've completed the journal.

| ✓ Check if done | Day 1 | Day 2 | Day 3 | Day 4 | Day 5 | Day 6 | Day 7 | TOTALS |
|---|---|---|---|---|---|---|---|---|
| **WEEK 1 HABIT TRACKER** | | | | | | | | |
| **ADD 5 HABITS** | | | | | | | | |
| 1. Eat a healthy breakfast | | | | | | | | |
| 2. Eat vegetables and fruits | | | | | | | | |
| 3. Eat whole grains | | | | | | | | |
| 4. Eat healthy fats | | | | | | | | |
| 5. Move! | | | | | | | | |
| **BREAK 5 HABITS** | | | | | | | | |
| 1. No TV while eating | | | | | | | | |
| 2. No sugar | | | | | | | | |
| 3. No snacks | | | | | | | | |
| 4. Only moderate meat and dairy | | | | | | | | |
| 5. No eating at restaurants | | | | | | | | |
| **5 BONUS HABITS** | | | | | | | | |
| 1. Keep diet records | | | | | | | | |
| 2. Keep exercise/activity records | | | | | | | | |
| 3. Move more! | | | | | | | | |
| 4. Eat "real" food | | | | | | | | |
| 5. Write your daily goals | | | | | | | | |
| **Totals** | | | | | | | | |

**DIRECTIONS:**

1. At the end of each day, check off which Add, Break and Bonus habits you have completed.
2. At the end of the week, total the columns and the rows to see how you've progressed.

| WEEK 2 HABIT TRACKER | | | | | | | |
|---|---|---|---|---|---|---|---|
| Day 8 | Day 9 | Day 10 | Day 11 | Day 12 | Day 13 | Day 14 | TOTALS |
| **ADD 5 HABITS** | | | | | | | |
| | | | | | | | |
| | | | | | | | |
| | | | | | | | |
| | | | | | | | |
| | | | | | | | |
| **BREAK 5 HABITS** | | | | | | | |
| | | | | | | | |
| | | | | | | | |
| | | | | | | | |
| | | | | | | | |
| | | | | | | | |
| **5 BONUS HABITS** | | | | | | | |
| | | | | | | | |
| | | | | | | | |
| | | | | | | | |
| | | | | | | | |
| | | | | | | | |

# HABIT TRACKER

**REMINDER:**

Total the columns and rows of your Habit Tracker to see which habits you're having success with and which are a problem for you.

See pages 58-59 of The Mayo Clinic Diet.

WEEK 1 HABIT T

| ✓ Check if done | Day 1 | Day 2 | Day |
|---|---|---|---|
| **ADD 5 HABITS** | | | |
| 1. Eat a healthy breakfast | ✓ | ✓ | |
| 2. Eat vegetables and fruits | ✓ | ✓ | ✓ |
| 3. Eat whole grains | ✓ | ✓ | ✓ |
| 4. Eat healthy fats | ✓ | ✓ | |
| 5. Move! | ✓ | | |
| **BREAK 5 HABITS** | | | |
| 1. No TV while eating | | | |
| 2. No sugar | | ✓ | ✓ |
| 3. No snacks | | ✓ | ✓ |
| 4. Only moderate meat and dairy | ✓ | ✓ | |
| 5. No eating at restaurants | ✓ | ✓ | |
| **5 BONUS HABITS** | | | |

The sample above demonstrates how to fill out your Habit Tracker.

# Lose It!

**TODAY'S GOAL:**

**TODAY'S ACTIVITIES:**     🕐 Time

|  |  |
|---|---|
|  |  |
|  |  |
|  |  |
|  |  |

| Total time (in minutes) |  |
|---|---|

**TODAY'S DATE**

**REMINDER:**
Remember to weigh yourself at the end of each week.

**WHAT I ATE TODAY:**

| 🕐 Time | Food item | Amount |
|---|---|---|
|  |  |  |
|  |  |  |
|  |  |  |
|  |  |  |
|  |  |  |
|  |  |  |
|  |  |  |
|  |  |  |
|  |  |  |
|  |  |  |
|  |  |  |

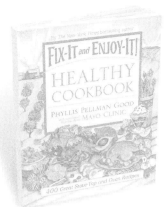

# 400 quick, healthy and delicious recipes

— from *The New York Times* best-selling cookbook author Phyllis Pellman Good and Mayo Clinic!

Discover the best of both worlds — easy and delicious recipes with special attention to health benefits. Each and every one of the 400 recipes in this book relies heavily on ingredients that are rich in nutrients considered to promote health and prevent disease. Plus, each recipe has been analyzed by Mayo Clinic dietitians for nutritional value and adapted to fit within the *Mayo Clinic Healthy Weight Pyramid.*

# The last diet you'll ever need!

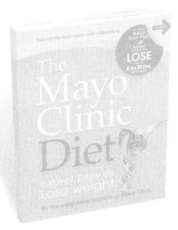

*The Mayo Clinic Diet* is based upon years of knowledge in working with patients to control their weight. Begin your journey to a healthy weight and all of the benefits that brings to you. Follow *The Mayo Clinic Diet!*

To learn more about Mayo Clinic health information products, go to

**Bookstore.MayoClinic.com.**

To learn more about Good Books publishing, go to

**GoodBooks.com.**

When you purchase Mayo Clinic books, DVDs and newsletters, proceeds are used to further medical education and research at Mayo Clinic.

# For the Better Health
## of every woman ...

### GET TWO FREE GIFTS WHEN YOU TRY
### *MAYO CLINIC WOMEN'S HEALTHSOURCE*

**Mayo Clinic has devoted an entire newsletter to bringing women the important information they need to take control of their health and their lives. Try it today and get two FREE Special Reports — "must reading" for every woman over 50.**

**MAYO CLINIC
WOMEN'S HEALTHSOURCE**

**WEIGHT CONTROL**
WHAT WORKS AND WHY

**JOINT HEALTH**
KEEP YOUR JOINTS MOVING
THROUGH LIFE

*Weight Control* will help you prevent the effects of obesity and lower your risk of breast and uterine cancer, diabetes and stroke.

*Joint Health* brings you the latest, best advice from Mayo Clinic specialists on protecting your joints from damage, remaining flexible and living pain-free.

Get both reports as free gifts when you try *Mayo Clinic Women's HealthSource.*

Each issue helps you do the things today that will set the stage for a healthier future. Get the latest, Mayo Clinic-approved ways to avoid, reduce or treat heart disease ... osteoporosis ... diabetes ... fibromyalgia ... arthritis ... the effects of aging on your skin ... decline in vision and hearing ... and much more.

The first issue is yours on a free-trial basis, and the two Special Reports are yours as our gifts, no matter what.

Order by visiting us at Bookstore.MayoClinic.com and clicking Women's HealthSource.

Mayo Clinic wants every woman to enjoy good health at any age. Try an issue of *Mayo Clinic Women's HealthSource* and discover the value of reliable health information every month.

## Visit *Mayo Clinic Women's HealthSource* at
## Bookstore.MayoClinic.com
## to learn more about this free-gift offer.

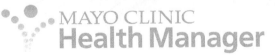

# MAYO CLINIC
## Health Manager

Powered by Microsoft® HealthVault™

## A new way to protect and manage your family's health

### Helping you do what you do best ... protect your family's health

▶ Store and manage health information online.
▶ Receive individualized health recommendations for each member of your family.
▶ Use customized trackers for various symptoms and conditions.

For more information visit *www.MayoClinic.com*.

I decided to go to Mayo Clinic.

*It was like nothing I'd ever seen before. The doctors are true specialists and the personal care is amazing. I wish that I'd gone there first. My answer was Mayo Clinic.*

MICHELLE FRITS
Lake in the Hills, Illinois

For more than 100 years, people from all walks of life have found answers at Mayo Clinic. We work with many insurance companies and are an in-network provider for millions of people. To make an appointment, please visit *www.MayoClinic.org*. In most cases, a physician referral is not needed.

ROCHESTER,        JACKSONVILLE,      SCOTTSDALE & PHOENIX,
MINNESOTA         FLORIDA            ARIZONA

## MAYO CLINIC